CW01653380

Breast is Best

Penny and Andrew Stanway are London-trained doctors who were married in 1969. They have two children, both of whom were breast fed.

Penny Stanway has spent some time in general practice and in research but it was during her appointment as Senior Medical Officer to a large Area Health Authority that she found there was a need for an up-to-date book about breast feeding. She is particularly interested in the prevention of childhood diseases and answers readers' letters in a well-known magazine for parents.

Andrew Stanway was a medical registrar at a London teaching hospital until six years ago. He now lectures, broadcasts, writes and makes films on medical topics both for the medical and dental professions and for the general public. Andrew Stanway has written several books including *Taking the Rough with the Smooth* (Pan Books, 1976) about dietary fibre, *Pears Encyclopedia* and *Encyclopedia of Alternative Medicine*.

Also published by Andrew Stanway in Pan Books
Taking the Rough with the Smooth

Penny and Andrew Stanway

Breast is Best

a common sense approach to breast feeding

Foreword by Dr Hugh Jolly MA MD FRCP DCH

Pan Original Pan Books London and Sydney

for Susanna and Amy

First published 1978 by Pan Books Ltd,
Cavaye Place, London SW10 9PG
5th printing 1980
© Penny and Andrew Stanway 1978
Foreword © Hugh Jolly 1978
ISBN 0 330 26193 2
Printed and bound in Great Britain by
Richard Clay (The Chaucer Press) Ltd, Bungay, Suffolk

This book is sold subject to the condition that it shall not, by way of trade or otherwise, be lent, re-sold, hired out or otherwise circulated without the publisher's prior consent in any form of binding or cover other than that in which it is published and without a similar condition including this condition being imposed on the subsequent purchaser

Acknowledgements We should like to thank the following who gave us valuable help in checking through the manuscript at its final stage and offering us the benefit of their very considerable experience: Dr Katherine Elliott, Assistant Director, The Ciba Foundation; La Leche League of Great Britain; Angela Helszajn, Secretary of the Breast feeding Promotion Group of the National Childbirth Trust, and Dr Frank Hytten. Our thanks are especially due to Dr Hugh Jolly, who gave us valuable help and advice and also wrote the Foreword

Contents

Some useful addresses

La Leche League of Great Britain, BM 3424, London WC1V 6XX. Mail should be addressed to the central office but personal telephone calls should be made to Cambridge (0223) 311291

National Childbirth Trust, 9 Queensborough Terrace, London W2 3TB
telephone 01–229 9319

For Egnell Pump hire contact National Childbirth Trust for local hiring point

Foreword

This book, while written for parents, should convince doctors and nurses as well as the parents themselves that there is a need for another book on breast feeding. Unfortunately, there is still serious ignorance amongst those whose task it is to advise mothers, with the result that they are bombarded by differing advice as to how to breast feed successfully. This is not due to changes in fads and fashions but to lack of training in the physiological processes of lactation which are so well set out in this book.

I started writing this foreword while working in the Middle East. I was appalled to hear young British midwives advising Arab mothers on breast feeding, describing methods which should have been discarded years ago. The clock has no part to play in breast feeding and yet these mothers were being told to feed three-hourly or four-hourly. This could have been correct if they had been veterinary surgeons advising farmers about the feeding of calves, but, because of the enormous differences in the composition of cows' milk compared with human milk and in the very growth processes of babies and calves, was totally incorrect for human mothers. I also keep hearing the appalling advice to feed 'ten minutes each side'. Whoever first invented that catchphrase had no knowledge of the physiology of lactation.

Fortunately, all this is explained here in a straightforward and understandable manner. As the authors describe the latest information on the difference between human milk and cows' milk, one is left with the nightmare this must mean for the manufacturers of cows' milk preparations. Their present attempts to modify cows' milk cannot hope to keep up with the advances in our understanding of the composition of human milk. One can only pity them their impossible task as they dismantle and convert their manufacturing plants.

On the other hand, one is left feeling an enormous relief for today's mothers who have no need to worry about the problems raised by feeding cows' milk to their babies. In fact, the more that is discovered about breast milk the more incredible it seems that we ever stopped using it.

It is so important for mothers to realize that failure to breast feed results from lack of the right sort of help rather than from their genes. There is so much more to breast feeding than just getting food into the baby, but it is not difficult to achieve if the atmosphere is right. My most enjoyable hospital work in the week is the morning's round in the maternity ward where I sit in turn on each new mother's bed and talk with her and her husband about breast feeding.

I warmly recommend the Stanways' book to all mothers. They will not only learn the enormous advantages to themselves and their babies from breast feeding, but will be armoured against the ignorant 'advice' which every breast feeding mother still has to face.

Hugh Jolly

Preface

'Why a book about breast feeding? Surely it's the most natural thing in the world . . . you don't need to learn about it.'

This is typical of the response we had when we told doctors and lay people alike that we were writing this book. But if it *is* so natural to breast feed it would be interesting to know why so many women in the Western world simply can't do it.

The answer is that it *is* natural but the ability to do it successfully doesn't necessarily come naturally. If you find this hard to believe, just bear in mind that less than a quarter of week-old babies in the USA are being breast fed and that at six months the figure has fallen to 5 per cent. In the UK about 50 to 60 per cent of women are breast feeding when they leave hospital (although the level in some hospitals is higher) but about a third of these will already have stopped by one month. To those mothers who find breast feeding easy, a book such as this may seem a complete waste of time but we hope it will be a help to those who don't.

Of all the phases in a woman's reproductive life, lactation has been the least understood and the most debased. At a time when we know more about female sexuality and reproductive life than ever, there is still appalling ignorance about breast feeding. Unfortunately, this ignorance spreads right through the medical and nursing professions and so makes it very difficult for today's mother to know where to turn for good advice. This has been made even more difficult because medical advice itself has changed so often.

What we have aimed to do is to clarify this confusion and in so doing to cut away all the 'mumsy' talk so often associated with breast feeding advice. This isn't because we're hard or cynical about the emotional and spiritual bonds that exist between a mother and her child but rather because experience has taught us that today's mother wants facts and straight talking. For this reason you'll find that there are areas in which we have been very brief: we have made an effort not to fill the book with theories and suppositions, not to mention the old wives' tales that abound elsewhere!

In order to help the reader learn how to breast feed successfully and cope with any problems, we've screened the world's literature, drawn evidence from a large number of medical journals and talked to experts with a wealth of experience in three continents. Most important though, we've listened to mothers.

This is not a 'roses round the door' book to make women feel they ought to breast feed even if they don't want to. No one has the right to do that. We have, however, presented the evidence in favour of breast feeding in a way that even the most sceptical or half-hearted mother should find acceptable.

Some people consider breast feeding to be unimportant today because of the practical alternative available, while others think that it is an essential part of good mothering. Both views are, of course, extreme but it's surprising how difficult it is to discuss breast feeding because the whole subject has become such an emotional one.

If you want to breast feed – or help somebody else to – read on. Millions of women the world over cope perfectly well . . . we in the West have simply lost the knack.

Dr Penny Stanway MB BS LRCP MRCS
Dr Andrew Stanway MB MRCP

1 So you want to breast feed

'Why on earth should I need a book to teach me how to breast feed?' we can hear you saying. 'Haven't women fed their babies for thousands of years? And how do all the millions of women in underdeveloped countries get on – they all breast feed and they don't learn from books?'

The answer is more complex than it seems, as any failed breast feeding mother will know. We live in a society in which breast feeding has become unfashionable and at a time when most young mothers go into pregnancy never having seen anyone breast feeding. Because breast feeding has fallen from grace in the eyes of modern women (and men), it no longer comes instinctively to many mothers and has to be learnt just like any other skill. In fact, breast feeding probably never has been entirely instinctive, but in the past other women helped and taught the new breast feeding mother and so ensured that breast feeding was almost universally successful. Evidence from many parts of the world has shown that in the past, babies of women who failed to produce enough milk simply died. This alone was an enormous incentive for women to help each other to make a success of breast feeding – as indeed they nearly all did.

Your baby won't need teaching how to feed – that's a natural instinct – but we're a long way from natural instincts so far as the mother's role is concerned today. Most mothers need help and encouragement if they are to succeed.

Before we go any further, let's get one thing straight. With the right advice and encouragement almost every woman can breast feed happily and successfully for as long as she and her baby want. In a campaign to encourage and support breast feeding in

Minneapolis, 96 per cent of nearly 3,000 women were fully breast feeding at two months, and 84 per cent were still breast feeding at six. But don't think that this is in any way typical of the USA, which is said to have the lowest breast feeding rate in the world. Fewer than 25 per cent of babies ever receive breast milk and in many hospitals no babies breast feed at all. Yet as recently as 1916, 60 per cent of women in the USA were still breast feeding their babies at one year.

Why then do so many mothers find breast feeding difficult, unacceptable or even downright distressing?

Man has been on the face of the earth for about a million years yet he has only reared milk-producing animals for the last 10,000 or so of these years. Only in the last fifty years has cows' milk (as a source of infant food) become anything like widespread. The unnatural change in diet from breast milk to cows' milk at so crucial a period in our lives is a modern intervention without parallel in the history of mankind. So massive and uncontrolled a change is it that it has led one researcher in the field to call it 'the greatest uncontrolled trial ever to have been done on human beings'. Man has become strangely obsessed with cows' milk and this obsession ought to be seriously questioned. The trouble is that in the West the advertising industry has made cows' milk into a food with almost magical properties and the milkman into some sort of folk hero. Could it be that this over-emphasis in adult life on the goodness of cows' milk is closely tied (albeit subconsciously) to the fact that we deprive our babies of the very milk they should be getting – their mothers' milk?

Why should all this be worrying to the woman who has decided to breast feed? Today, if a mother has any problems with her milk supply, she is immediately handicapped further by a sense of guilt and personal failure. Then, because cows' milk feeds are so readily available with little fear of personal failure attached she soon starts her baby on the bottle.

The sad part of all this is that breast feeding is still considered by most people to be simply a way of getting food into a baby. In reality it is so much more. Many women who feel that breast feeding isn't for them, or who seriously question why it is that so many Western women fail to breast feed, assume that they cannot do so for perfectly good biological reasons. They assume that because bottle feeding has been practised for so long, modern woman has become biologically incapable of producing enough milk.

The truth of the matter is that as recently as the beginning of this century the majority of babies in the Western world were fed at the breast and as far as medical science is aware it would take many generations for such a radical biological change to take place – not a mere seventy years. The final condemnation of this argument comes when these so-called 'genetically incapable' women get help and encouragement and go on to feed their babies successfully. Most women fail to breast feed because of their environment, not because of their genes.

A study in France showed that the numbers of babies getting *no* breast milk at all rose from 31 per cent to 51 per cent in a matter of five years and over a period of twenty years in Bristol the number of three-month-olds breast feeding fell from 74 per cent to 36 per cent. These falls are so large and occurred so quickly that no genetic explanation could possibly be acceptable. It had to be an environmental change – a change in attitude.

The crunch came as new facts about the disadvantages of even the newest 'modified' cows' milks came to light. Cows' milk preparations were found to lack Vitamin B6, Vitamin E and linoleic acid; to be too high in protein, sodium and phosphorus and to cap it all it was found that there were many more protective antibodies against disease in breast milk than had ever been thought. The discovery was also made that a baby's gut wall could leak whole protein molecules from cows' milk into the bloodstream, and that these 'foreign' proteins could lay the foundation for eczema and asthma both in infancy and in later life.

Baby milk manufacturers speedily changed their formulae to keep pace with these new discoveries and there was talk about vaccinating herds of specially bred cows to give them immunity against human diseases. But by this time the damage had been done and when mothers demanded that they should be allowed to feed their babies with the best baby food of all, they found that the art of breast feeding had been all but lost. Mothers had lost confidence in their natural ability and common sense and professionals (midwives, doctors and health visitors) had seen few mothers successfully breast feeding and had been brainwashed by rigid advice on schedules for breast feeding. Hospitals had forgotten that they existed to do their best for the patients and not to idolize the new god, 'routine', and even the mothers' own mothers were often of little help as they were among the first to use the new, magic cows' milk when they fed their children.

So this is where we came in. We have found as parents, health educators and doctors that few mothers can get good and consistent advice about breast feeding. If they can, it tends to stop as soon as they appear to be managing on their own at home. The trouble is that while the new mother might like the idea of breast feeding, as soon as any problem – however small – crops up, she is lucky if she can continue, because she will be showered with differing advice from all sides. This is especially upsetting as she will probably feel unable to stand up to any upset or to sort out conflicting advice so soon after childbirth. Once she's put the baby on the bottle, she'll feel depressed and guilty. Indeed, many women experience a deep and lasting sense of failure should this occur.

Why you'll need help

Today's society isn't geared to helping its young mothers breast feed, even when they want to. For a start, it's 'normal' for babies to be bottle fed and if you breast feed you'll be 'abnormal'. You've got to be prepared for that. Even the 'token breast feeder' we describe later will not understand the mother who believes in natural breast feeding. Though more mothers start to breast feed their babies now, the vast majority of babies are soon completely or almost completely bottle fed. Statistics show that by three months 70 per cent of breast fed babies will have had bottles and solid foods – and that's the so-called 'breast fed babies'! Mothers who totally and solely breast feed their babies are rare.

A girl can reach motherhood without ever having seen a baby at the breast. Breast feeding will rarely have been mentioned at school, even in Biology and Sex Education classes. Her friends and relatives will be far more familiar with bottle feeding and while not actively discouraging her from breast feeding, they will make a very good job of persuading the mother-to-be that a bottle fed baby will be as contented and healthy as a breast-fed one.

Perhaps more insidious is the fact that today's young woman is brought up and educated to think of herself as a wage-earner and career woman. When she marries, her income will almost certainly be necessary to start a home and it's difficult for her to think of giving this up when a baby comes along. She tends to tell herself that she may go back to work part-time soon after the baby is born, or perhaps just a little later. She may even organize things so that she can keep her job and just take maternity leave. In any event, she's not thinking of herself in relation to her baby but rather of her role in relation to her husband and job.

It's often said that today's mother doesn't breast feed because she has to go back to work so soon. The fact is that only a small percentage of women actually go back to work while their children are young. What a shame they can't admit to themselves that they will be unlikely to go back in the short term and just relax and look forward to being a mother.

But more mothers are showing an interest in breast feeding today. Unfortunately, their success rates are poor and most of them put this down to 'not having enough milk'. This is completely wrong as has been shown in studies all over the world. There are very few women who cannot breast feed if they want to and if they are given enough help.

At this point some readers will be shaking their heads and saying that there is already a lot of help available to the pregnant and nursing mother. This is simply not true. There are lots of professional people employed by the National Health Service who can and do advise mothers but a large amount of their advice is frankly unhelpful and is often contradictory anyway. Why should this be? It's mainly because doctors, nurses and midwives are influenced by society and fashion just like the rest of us. They have also been brainwashed over the last forty years or so into believing that cows' milk really is the equal of breast milk. Two recent studies in England bear this out. In one, 355 women were asked what advice they had had during pregnancy about feeding their babies. Three out of four women had had no positive advice to breast feed and 5 per cent were actually recommended to bottle feed. The second survey found that 81 per cent of women had received no encouragement whatsoever ante-natally to breast feed.

We have found that most doctors pay lip service to breast feeding but won't go all out to convince mothers it's the very best thing. A survey of American paediatricians showed that they advised mothers according to the breast feeding experience of their own wives. If their wives had had a difficult time or were unsuccessful then they legislated for difficulties with their patients and so put them off breast feeding. A distinguished American paediatrician once lectured fellow paediatricians on infant feeding in New York. When by the end of his oration he still had not mentioned breast feeding, one of the delegates asked why. The paediatrician answered that he never recommended breast feeding because it was too difficult!

What help is there?

Pregnant women are often overwhelmed with help and advice from friends, relatives, neighbours and ante-natal classes where one lesson on infant feeding is usually included. The doctor or midwife looking after the expectant mother may ask how she is going to feed her baby and may proffer some advice and even examine her breasts. When the baby is born, the hospital or district midwife, together with the doctor (family doctor or clinic doctor), health visitor, friends, relatives and neighbours, will again offer advice about feeding the baby.

But although there may be masses of lay and professional 'help' and 'advice', because most people today have forgotten how to practise the art of successful breast feeding, let alone how to teach it, such help may be of little or no value. It is exactly because of this confusion that self-help organizations came into being. Mothers came to realize that the only people who seemed to know what they were doing were other mothers who had successfully breast fed their babies.

The National Childbirth Trust Breastfeeding Promotion Group is a self-help group which has organized a network of young mothers throughout the country who have breast fed their children and have been trained as breast feeding counsellors. They will help on the phone if you have problems and visit you at home if necessary. Also, La Leche League, an international organization, has recently started up in this country. Its various groups hold meetings and discussions about breast feeding and its group leaders will give help on the phone when necessary.

Both these organizations will help when needed. Should you have a problem with breast feeding, you won't want to wait to make an appointment to see your GP or clinic doctor and even your health visitor may be difficult to get hold of. You need help there and then, before you give the baby that first bottle.

Breast feeding isn't always as easy as falling off a log, contrary to what many successful mothers will tell you. There's nothing more annoying than having to listen to breast feeders telling you how easy it was (and by implication what a failure you are if you failed). We don't think breast feeding is necessarily easy – it's often a lot harder than most women expect – especially in the early days.

If all else fails you can teach yourself how to cope successfully with problems and we'll show you how.

2 How breast feeding works

This chapter and the next will give you an idea of how breast feeding works and why breast milk is the best for your baby. The practical details of breast feeding start in chapter 6 but the next few chapters fill in the essential background knowledge you'll need to understand how to breast feed and why things can go wrong. They'll bring you right up to date with all the major research carried out into breast feeding over the last twenty years or so. It's a terrible indictment of modern medicine that although a great deal of this key research has been published for years, most doctors and nurses are unaware of it.

Let's start by looking at the breasts themselves.

The breasts

A year or so before a girl's periods start, changes in the shape and size of her breasts, nipples and areolae begin and they carry on changing until her late teens. After this they remain the same until she becomes pregnant. Man is the only mammal in which the breasts enlarge before pregnancy. Breasts have also taken on a sexual role in courtship that isn't seen in other mammals and it's this that helps colour our attitudes to breast feeding in the Western world.

The lactating breast is made up of fifteen to twenty segments, each containing glandular tissue leading to a main duct which opens at the nipple. This means that there are between fifteen and twenty ducts opening on the nipple. You can see these openings as little crevices and if you stop for a moment when you're feeding your baby, you'll see drops of milk coming from them. Sometimes you can see fine sprays of milk coming from several ducts at a time.

In the pregnant or breast feeding woman the glandular part of each segment of the breast is rather like a bunch of grapes on a stalk which is the milk duct. Each 'grape' is called an alveolus or milk gland and has a tiny duct leading to the 'stalk' or main duct. The milk gland is lined with milk-producing cells, each bordering on the little duct, so that milk produced by these cells goes from the small to large duct and thence to the nipple. Around each milk gland is a network of branching, star-like muscle cells (myo-epithelial cells) which can contract, so squeezing the milk gland and forcing milk from the cells into the ducts.

The main duct from each segment of the breast widens as it comes under the areola and is capable of further distension as it fills with milk. This means that just beneath the areola there are fifteen to twenty milk 'reservoirs'. The diameter of each of these when full can be between half and one centimetre, so it's easy to see that a lot of milk can be stored ready for the baby at the beginning of each feed. These reservoirs are capable of storing even more milk after several weeks of breast feeding and some mothers notice that any leaking they may have had stops after six to eight weeks as their storage capacity increases.

The increase in size of the breasts during adolescence is caused by the laying down of fat and by the lengthening and branching of the milk ducts. At this stage there is no true glandular tissue but the formation of buds which will later develop into the milk glands is now begun. All these changes are controlled by the menstrual hormones.

During pregnancy many women notice tingling and fullness of their breasts as early as their first missed period. Indeed, breast sensations are often the first symptom of pregnancy. Little prominences around the areolae called Montgomery's tubercles become more noticeable at about six weeks and by five months most women find they need a larger bra. In a first pregnancy, the nipples and areolae begin to darken now. If you lose your baby at any time after five months, you'll lactate just as if you had given birth at full term. All these changes are caused by hormones (some of which are only present in pregnancy) circulating in the blood. On average, each breast weighs one and a half pounds more at the end of pregnancy, mainly because of the development of glandular tissue and the proliferation of the milk ducts.

The size of your breasts before pregnancy will have no bearing on your ability to breast feed because some small breasts actually contain more milk-producing glands than larger ones. It's the *increase* in the size of your breasts during pregnancy that is a good indicator of your ability to feed easily. As a general rule, if you need a bra one or two sizes larger by the end of pregnancy, you should have little trouble getting off to a good start. It has been found that the younger a woman is when she has her first pregnancy, the greater the increase in size of her breasts. This may explain why it is that in women having their first babies, younger ones tend to produce more milk than older ones at first. Women with very small breasts may be at a slight disadvantage early on, though, because their breasts can become overfilled more quickly than larger breasts and so either leak or have to be offered to the baby more frequently. As their storage capacity increases over the first few weeks this becomes less of a problem.

While we're on the subject of breast size, it's interesting to note that mothers often comment on the size of their babies' breasts. Newborn babies often have enlarged breasts. This is because of maternal hormones travelling across the placenta before birth. Sometimes milk even comes out of a baby's breasts. This is often called witches' milk and is seen both in boys and girls. The treatment is to ignore it – it will eventually disappear.

Not only do a woman's nipples become larger during pregnancy but they also become more 'protractile' – and so easier for the baby to take hold of with his mouth. There are a few women whose nipples don't change like this and their babies may have problems in 'latching on' at first. Details of how to overcome this problem can be found on page 93.

Milk production

Production of milk by the milk glands is under the influence of the hormones prolactin, growth hormone, the corticosteroids, thyroxine and insulin. Each milk gland is surrounded by a fine network of blood vessels and it is through this blood supply that the hormones reach the milk-producing cells. Blood also provides the materials from which milk is actually made by the cells.

Prolactin is the main milk-producing hormone and appears from the eighth week of pregnancy onwards, reaching its peak with the birth of the baby. It is prevented from producing milk in any volume during pregnancy by the high levels of oestrogen made by the placenta. After the baby is born and with the loss of the placenta, the oestrogen 'brakes' are removed and prolactin starts milk production in earnest. This usually occurs between the second and fourth days. The milk can come in earlier in women feeding their babies frequently and in those having their second or subsequent babies. Usually the milk comes in slowly but it may come in a deluge. This is quite normal, so don't let it worry you. The way to cope with it is to let your baby feed as often as you need to keep you comfortable.

Prolactin, the hormone that 'turns on the taps', is produced by the pituitary gland in the brain. The most important factor in the continued release of prolactin is nipple stimulation which sends nervous impulses to the pituitary. The holding and squeezing of the nipple and areola by the baby's mouth is more important than his *sucking*. Suckling increases the mother's prolactin which in turn increases her milk supply, so the more the baby feeds, the more milk is produced. Prolactin levels fluctuate throughout the day and are highest at night, even in non-lactating women.

As milk is produced by the milk glands, it is secreted into the milk ducts. We've already seen that the parts of the ducts under the areolae are capable of storing milk and an hour or so after a feed a third of the volume of milk making up a normal feed is already waiting in these distended ducts. This milk, known as foremilk, is low in fat content and hence in calories. Every woman produces milk after childbirth and so will have foremilk available for her baby whenever he wants to feed. However, the bulk of the milk is only supplied if the *let-down reflex* operates.

Getting milk into a baby in large enough amounts is a skill that needs to be learnt but like most skills it's acquired all the more quickly if you know the mechanisms involved. There are two vital mechanisms: one is the let-down reflex we've just mentioned and the other is the law of *supply and demand.*

The let-down reflex

After a feed, the milk-producing cells gradually enlarge, becoming round and full as they produce more milk. The fullness and slight lumpiness you may feel some time after a feed is caused by these swollen milk glands with their laden cells and ducts.

The milk in the cells can be forced into the ducts very quickly by the contraction of the muscle cells surrounding each milk gland and when this happens the milk is said to have been let down. This is the only way in which the baby can get this milk – without the let-down, the milk stays in the milk glands.

With the let-down, milk is pushed into the ducts so quickly that it sprays or drips from the nipples. This occurs in a series of spurts with a gap between each.

Milk produced by the let-down is known as hindmilk and makes up about two thirds of the milk available for a feed. Hindmilk is rich in calories and fat and without it a baby will not get enough milk to thrive. Foremilk contains 1.5 calories/ounce and hindmilk 30 calories/ounce. We don't as yet know for sure why this difference in fat content occurs.

The reason that many women fail to breast feed successfully is that their let-down reflex is faulty. This reflex is a delicately balanced mechanism, especially in the early weeks after childbirth when external factors can prevent its satisfactory development and action. When you hear people talking about the 'establishment' of breast feeding, they are really talking about the establishment of a satisfactory, reliable, well-conditioned let-down reflex. Until the let-down reflex is well and truly established, you can't be sure you are going to breast feed successfully.

So how does this all-important reflex work? The main factor involved is the stimulation of the skin of the nipple and the tissues under the areola which normally occurs when the baby feeds at the breast. This is the same stimulus that causes prolactin release. Nervous impulses travel from the nipple to the pituitary gland and cause the release of another hormone – oxytocin – into the blood. Oxytocin is taken in the blood to the breast and makes the muscle cells around the milk glands squeeze milk into the ducts. This cycle of suckling – nervous messages to the pituitary – oxytocin release – contraction of muscle cells with the subsequent release of milk into the ducts is what is known as the let-down reflex.

The time taken for the let-down reflex to work varies from woman to woman and in any one woman it can vary from day to day according to her surroundings, emotional state and other factors. When a baby is put to the breast the let-down takes a minimum of thirty to fifty seconds to work but it often takes longer than this and it can take two to three minutes for the maximum milk flow to be produced.

This means that a hungry baby may have finished all the available foremilk before the hindmilk has been let down and this delay can make him frustrated. Such frustration can worry the inexperienced mother to such an extent that she doesn't let down her milk at all. The let-down is such a delicate mechanism that many strong emotions such as fear, worry and embarrassment can prevent its action.

Nipple stimulation is not the only way in which the milk can be let down – the reflex is easily conditioned by other stimuli. The sight or sound of your baby (or even someone else's baby) can suddenly let down your milk, particularly if you haven't fed for some time. Some women find that as they prepare to feed their babies, their let-down works before suckling is begun at all, simply because the reflex has been conditioned by their routine. This is a good thing because the baby then doesn't have to wait for the milk to flow.

Besides causing the let-down, oxytocin has other effects. The uterus is sensitive to oxytocin and may contract when there is an increased level in the blood. The uterine contractions are rhythmical and are the cause of the 'afterpains' some mothers feel while feeding in the first few days. Also, while the milk is being let down, the breasts may tingle and feel tense. The let-down is usually a pleasant feeling for the mother and has been described as 'something between a sneeze and an orgasm'.

At the same time as the milk is let down, the skin of the breasts feels warmer to the touch than usual. In the early days of feeding it's easy to know when your let-down reflex is working because of the sensations in the breasts, leaking of milk from the breasts, the warmth of the breast skin and the contractions of the womb. Some mothers have none of these sensations yet have a very good let-down reflex – and any given woman may experience different let-down sensations from baby to baby.

Leaking. Warmth from a hot bath or from your baby's mouth can cause an initial leaking of milk without a true let-down. This is because there are contractile muscle fibres in the nipple and areola which are normally held contracted, so keeping the ducts closed. Warmth lengthens these fibres and releases their tight hold on the ducts, allowing milk to escape.

So far we've only considered the milk-producing effects of the mother's hormones but they also have other effects. The hormones produced during lactation seem to give the breast feeding mother a special feeling of happiness and joy. Animal research has shown that lactating rats are actually buffered against stressful situations by their hormones and it's quite possible that this may also be true in humans. Some people go so far as to call prolactin the 'mothering hormone'.

So much for the production and let-down of milk but how does it actually get to the baby? There are many old wives' tales about suckling but the most common is that the baby has to suck to get milk. This is not so, although the baby certainly exerts some suction to keep the nipple and areola in his mouth and in so doing will suck in some milk. He gets the foremilk from the reservoirs under the areola by a 'milking' action of his jaws. The further he can draw the nipple and areola into his mouth, the better he'll be able to empty the reservoirs. This is why the 'protractility' of the nipples is so important. This milking action stimulates the let-down reflex which ejects milk from the nipple in fine jets so that all he has to do is swallow. You'll notice that your baby will take several gulps of milk in a row and then rest for a while, keeping the breast in his mouth, before taking more gulps. This is because the milk lets down in spurts with a gap between each spurt. If oxytocin levels in the blood are continuously monitored during a feed they can be seen to rise and fall in waves corresponding with the ejection of the milk.

Supply and demand. All the time a baby is feeding, the nipple and surrounding area are stimulated, so causing the pituitary gland to release prolactin and oxytocin. Since prolactin controls milk production it's easy to see that the more suckling there is, the more prolactin will be produced, which in turn produces more milk. Also, the more episodes of suckling there are, the more reliable the let-down reflex becomes. This is the basis of the second principle you need to understand – that of supply and demand. If those caring for new mothers understood this principle, there would be far fewer breast feeding failures.

'Supply and demand' is not really a very good term because demand produces the supply and not the other way round. The more feeds your baby 'asks for' and gets in a day, the greater the supply of milk there will be. This has been proven in many surveys. For instance, in one survey in Sheffield in 1952, demand fed babies gained weight faster than those fed according to a schedule, showing that their mothers were producing more milk by feeding more often.

There are no limits to the number of feeds you can give your baby – every time he asks, he should be fed. This doesn't mean to say, though, that you can only feed your baby when he asks for a feed. If you want to feed him because your breasts are full or simply because you want to for the pleasure it'll give you, do. *Natural breast feeding puts no rules or limits on suckling time* (see page 89).

Babies allowed to feed as often as they want take very variable numbers of feeds during the twenty-four hours. In the early days some babies may want feeding every hour or so and the greatest number of feeds often occurs on the fifth day after birth. In the Sheffield survey we've just mentioned, 29 per cent of babies fed on demand wanted eight feeds on the fifth day and 10 per cent wanted more than nine.

In a textbook for doctors published in 1906, when successful breast feeding was the norm, the following schedule of feeds was recommended:

First day	4 feeds
Second day	6 feeds
Rest of the first month	10 feeds
Second and third months	8 feeds
Fourth and fifth months	7 feeds
Sixth to eleventh months	6 feeds

This is a far cry from the schedules so often recommended for breast fed babies in hospitals today (every four hours for a large baby and every three hours for a small one). This sort of schedule produces notoriously poor results whereas the 1906 type was much more successful. *However, completely unrestricted, natural breast feeding, involving very frequent feeds in the early days, is best of all, and any schedule should be discarded.*

A survey in Africa throws interesting light on this subject. Researchers watched mothers sleeping with their babies over many nights to see how often the babies fed while their mothers slept. No baby went longer than twenty minutes without feeding! Contrast these lucky babies with Western babies who are usually rationed to one feed a night until their mothers' milk dries up completely.

Never compare your baby with that of your neighbour in the next bed. Each baby is unique and should be allowed to be so. Some settle into a routine of six feeds a day within a few weeks but this is certainly *not* a goal to be aimed for, it's just one of many patterns that your baby may adopt in time. A word of warning here – one leading authority in the UK has said that in her experience if a baby has five or fewer feeds in a day, the likelihood is that the mother's milk will have dried up in a month through lack of stimulation of the breasts. *However many feeds your baby wants, let him have them.*

The length of a feed is also a matter for the individual baby to decide and shouldn't be laid down by doctors, midwives or even mothers. The average feeding time at one breast is about ten minutes but there are many babies who get all they need in five minutes and many others who need twenty minutes or more at each breast before they are satisfied. Feeding times vary for several reasons. First, the let-down may be slow to work so the baby doesn't start getting hindmilk for two or three minutes. Second, some babies are much greedier than others, suck more strongly and so get all they need in a shorter time. Third, some babies – especially in the early days – may not be very alert and so will need to take their time over a feed. All these situations are discussed in more detail later.

It's important not to curtail the length of feeds in the first few days particularly, because it's all too easy to take the baby from the breast before the let-down has worked at all. Many hospitals insist on very short suckling times in the first few days to prevent sore nipples but as we'll see later this is a fallacious argument. Short suckling times often prevent or delay the establishment of successful lactation and are of absolutely no benefit for mother or baby.

Finally, a question often asked by mothers who don't want to breast feed is how can they dry up their milk. Today we know that there is no need for any drugs to do this. If a mother simply doesn't breast feed, her milk will dry up by itself. Oestrogens, once used to dry up milk, have side-effects such as venous thrombosis, and stopping the drugs often causes a rebound of milk production. The use of new drugs such as bromocriptine to dry up milk is not only unnecessary but also expensive!

One other advantage of not using drugs to dry up milk artificially is that if a mother changes her mind and decides to breast feed, it is very much easier for her to work up her milk supply than if it had been artificially suppressed.

So much for the breasts themselves – now let's look at the milk they produce.

3 Breast milk – the perfect food

Until very recently it was thought that the advantages of breast milk were few. To most medical and nursing students these advantages were usually summed up as follows:

1 it's at the right temperature
2 it contains exactly what a baby needs
3 it's bacteria-free
4 it comes in such cute containers; and
5 the cat can't get at it!

For years this was the sort of level on which doctors and nurses were taught to consider breast milk. Small wonder then that when the baby milk manufacturers came up with their modified, 'improved' milks, both mothers and the medical profession thought they were getting something every bit as good as breast milk – and perhaps even better.

The outstanding characteristic of mammals is that they suckle or feed their young with their milk at least until they can get their own food. As mammals are so different from one another, it's not surprising that the milk they produce differs too. If an elephant, a rat, a sheep, a whale and a human all ate similar diets, it might be reasonable to expect that the milk they produce for their young would be similar. But of course they don't and their milks are correspondingly different. Over scores of thousands of years each mammal has developed a milk to suit its own young. This milk takes into account the animal's rate of growth, type of digestive tract, natural illnesses and many other factors.

The basic similarity that runs through all milks, though, is that they are made up of the same groups of substances: water, proteins, fats, carbohydrates, minerals, vitamins and anti-infective substances. The differences occur because these substances are present in different amounts and in varying proportions. On top of this, these seven things are not single entities (apart from water) but are often made up of whole families of substances, each one different from the next. For example, there are many different sorts of proteins, some of which differ from woman to woman, let alone between woman and cow!

When we look at whale milk we find it has a very high fat content, which in turn gives it a very high calorie content. (It is in fact richer than double cream.) This is essential because the infant whale has to form a layer of thick blubber very quickly so as to protect it from the cold water. The protein content of rabbit's milk is very high compared with human milk. It contains 14 per cent protein compared with the 1.2 per cent in human milk. This is necessary because the growth rate of the young rabbit is so fast. (A rabbit doubles its birth weight in six days, whereas a human baby takes about 140 days.) High milk protein levels are a must for every newborn animal that grows quickly, because protein provides the basic building blocks for the growth of body tissues. Compared with most other mammalian young, human babies grow very slowly and breast milk has a correspondingly lower level of protein.

Over the years there have been reports of mammals taking the young of other species into their care and feeding them but this is very unusual. The first time one group of mammals used another's milk to any great extent was when humans started to give their babies cows' milk this century. Of course, over the centuries the occasional baby had been reared on the milk of another animal (Romulus and Remus were supposedly reared by a wolf) but on the whole the use of cows' milk is a new phenomenon. Before this century if a mother didn't want to feed her baby, another woman had to take over if the baby was to have a good chance of surviving and in some countries even today a baby will die if the mother doesn't feed it herself.

Why did we choose cows' milk as our breast milk substitute? It's a particularly good question because cows' milk is by no means the nearest in composition to human milk – donkey milk is much closer! People in other countries have used the milk from goats, donkeys, buffalo, sheep, llamas, reindeer, mares and camels for their babies over the years but the great move towards artificial feeding came from the West where herds of cows were already being reared for meat and dairy produce, so it seemed convenient and economically sensible to use cows' milk. Cows are also docile, easily herded animals that produce large volumes of milk from a given volume of grass. Add to this the fact that their four teats make for easy milking and it soon becomes obvious why we have tended to use cows as a source of milk.

The most obvious difference between cows' milk and breast milk is that cows' milk contains more protein and less sugar. This led doctors and food scientists to 'modify' it earlier this century so that it came to resemble breast milk more closely. They did this by diluting it and adding sugar. This basic modification was used for years and mothers either adapted liquid 'doorstep' milk by diluting it with water, adding sugar and boiling it, or they bought dried, evaporated or condensed milk and made up their own formula by adding water and sugar in the recommended amounts. Over the years we have come to realize that these basic modifications are not enough because of the many differences between the two milks. We now know that these differences can lead to medical problems in babies drinking cows' milk preparations and we'll consider some of these later.

What milk contains

Water

The liquid part of milk is water and all the other constituents are either dissolved or suspended in it, making it appear white, creamy or yellow, depending on the proportions of various substances present.

Water is vital for the existence of every cell in the body and a lack of it causes dehydration, cell damage and eventual death. Certain body cells are more susceptible than others to dehydration and brain cells are especially at risk. A dehydrated baby risks getting brain damage.

Breast milk is the perfect food for human babies because the proportions of water and the other constituents are just right. Many mothers worry that their milk might be too 'watery'. This is very unlikely and anyway there's nothing you can tell about the nutrient value of breast milk simply by looking at it. Yellowy breast milk is in no way superior to thin blue-white milk. Yellow breast milk is not comparable to 'rich, creamy cows' milk'. A thirsty baby given breast milk gets the right amount of water to satisfy his thirst. A breast fed baby need never be given water, provided he gets enough breast milk. In very hot weather the breast feeding *mother* should take more water, not the baby. On the other hand a baby drinking cows' milk is in danger of taking too high a proportion of the substances dissolved in the water because the concentrations of some of them are too high (even in modified cows' milk). This is especially likely to happen if he is already dehydrated from diarrhoea, vomiting or sweating from a fever. In addition to these unavoidable hazards mothers often make up milk feeds too strong, so reducing the proportion of liquid to solid. The baby gets too much solid, gets dehydrated and can become severely ill. Recent modifications of cows' milk preparations have put this right to some extent but the proportions of water and other substances are still by no means the same as those of breast milk and there's still a danger, especially in the early weeks of life.

The stools of bottle fed babies contain less water than those of breast fed babies and this is one reason why they get constipated more often.

Protein

About 1.2 per cent of breast milk is protein. This protein is made up of curd protein (casein) and the whey proteins (lactalbumin and lactoglobulin). Cows' milk has 3.3 per cent protein (a calf doubles its birth weight in fifty days) and this extra is composed of six times as much casein as there is in breast milk.

When milk enters a baby's stomach, it's turned into curds and whey. The curds are made of casein, so it's not surprising that the curds of cows' milk are much bulkier than those of breast milk. They are so tough and bulky that many babies get indigestion if they are given unmodified cows' milk to drink.

This is the main reason behind the basic 'modifications' of cows' milk – dilution with water. Adding water dilutes the tough, indigestible casein. Boiling, homogenization and the addition of various chemicals have also been used to alter the casein so as to make it less tough and indigestible.

Breast milk protein forms finely separated curds in the stomach which then pass quickly and easily through into the small intestine where they are easily broken down. This means that the stomach of a breast fed baby empties more quickly than that of a bottle fed baby and this is why he gets hungry more quickly and needs frequent feeds. Cows' milk curds stay in the stomach for about four hours. *So four-hourly feeding for a bottle fed baby is reasonable, but a breast fed baby will need feeding more often.*

A baby only uses about half the protein available in cows' milk, whilst a breast fed baby uses all the protein, with virtually no wastage. The protein a bottle fed baby doesn't use is partly passed out in the stools (which makes a bottle fed baby's stools bulkier than a breast fed baby's) and partly broken down before being excreted by the kidneys in the urine. Because there is so little wastage from breast milk, a baby has to drink less of it. This is why breast fed babies normally drink a much smaller volume than do bottle fed ones. Test weighing a breast fed baby can easily be misleading if this is forgotten – the amount a breast fed baby drinks should never be compared with the amount drunk by a bottle fed one. If you gauge the amount your breast fed baby has taken by test weighing, you'll almost certainly end up worrying unnecessarily.

The lactoglobulin fraction of milk protein contains highly specialized proteins – the immunoglobulins (IgA, IgD, IgE, IgG and IgM). These carry the antibodies against disease and recent research into these substances has revolutionized our thinking on breast milk. For years it was thought that a baby only obtained antibodies from its mother before birth across the placenta and that none were given via breast milk. That this was not the only method of antibody transfer in other mammals had been known for a long time. We now know that babies continue to receive these essential antibodies from their mothers' milk – assuming of course that they're breast fed! Colostrum, a special sort of milk produced in the first few days after birth, contains large amounts of lactoglobulin, so we can now say with complete assurance that colostrum is vitally important for the future health of a baby. Mature breast milk also contains antibodies but in smaller amounts than those in colostrum.

These milk antibodies are similar to those which the mother has in her blood and protect the baby against bacterial and viral illnesses from which the mother has suffered or has been immunized against. They can act locally in the baby's gut and can also be absorbed into his bloodstream through the gut lining. Among the illnesses that a baby can be protected from in this way are tetanus, whooping cough, pneumonia, diphtheria, *E. coli* gastroenteritis, typhoid, dysentery, 'flu and various other viral illnesses including polio. Quite a list! Later, a baby will manufacture his own antibodies in response to infection or immunization but during the first few months he can't and so has to get antibodies from his mother. This period of absent and then gradually increasing antibody formation by the baby has been called the 'immunity gap' and it's a gap that can only be filled by breast milk.

Immunoglobulin A (IgA) in the mother's colostrum and milk coats the lining of the baby's gut in the first few days after birth and prevents many infective organisms and other large protein molecules from entering the baby's bloodstream. When the baby begins to make his own IgA, the mother's becomes unnecessary but in the meantime this IgA coating prevents the development not only of some generalized infections but also of allergy to various foodstuffs in many babies. We'll talk about this more in chapter 4.

Cows' milk contains antibodies too but of course these are antibodies against cows' diseases, not human ones. In any case lactoglobulin (together with lactoferrin, another anti-infective agent) is altered to such an extent by the heating involved in the treatment of fresh cows' milk that it loses its antibody activity. So few cows' milk preparations available to human babies would contain active antibodies even if they were of any use! The ultimate irony is that calves reared on heat-treated milk or on dried milk powders get more enteritis than those drinking fresh untreated milk. This enteritis is effectively treated by giving them fresh cows' milk. The reason why even calves fare badly on treated cows' milk is that this treatment destroys the milk's antibody activity.

An interesting parallel to this was seen in a nursery in Belgrade where an epidemic of E. coli gastro-enteritis could not be stopped even when the babies were all fed with donated breast milk (boiled before use). Not until the breast milk was given fresh from the donors, with no boiling, was the epidemic controlled.

Besides protein in milk there are free amino acids and the proportions of these differ in human and cows' milk. Breast milk, for instance, contains more cystine compared with cows' milk which contains more of another amino acid known as methionine. This is especially important for premature babies because they are incapable of using methionine until they become more mature. It is also possible that the high levels of some amino acids found in the bottle fed baby's blood might in some circumstances damage the nervous system.

Nucleotides are building blocks necessary for protein manufacture (like the amino acids) and they are present in human milk in larger amounts than in cows' milk. More important perhaps is the fact that the main one found in cows' milk, orotic acid, is not found at all in human milk. More research needs to be done in this field before we know how important this is. But it raises a crucial question. Might there actually be substances in cows' milk that, although only present in tiny amounts, could be positively harmful to human babies?

Fat

The fat in milk is present both in saturated and unsaturated forms but breast milk contains a higher percentage of unsaturated fat. This has recently led some baby milk manufacturers to replace some of the fat in cows' milk with unsaturated vegetable oils in an attempt to make the milk more like breast milk. Their early efforts led to some dire consequences as linoleic acid (one of these unsaturated vegetable oils) was added in far greater quantities than are naturally present in human milk. Some babies suffered from a severe kind of anaemia as a result!

Whilst cows' milk contains less linoleic acid than breast milk, most baby milks available in this country contain enough to prevent the symptoms of deficiency (poor growth and thick, scaly skin) even without the substitution of vegetable oils.

As yet we don't know whether the unsaturated fat content of breast milk is in any way protective against heart disease. This is still a matter for speculation. We do know though that another essential body fat – cholesterol – is present in larger amounts in breast milk than in cows' milk. After all the scares surrounding cholesterol and heart attacks and the possible link between the two you might well ask whether a cholesterol-rich milk is best for babies.

Ironically, it looks as though these higher cholesterol levels somehow accustom breast fed babies to handling cholesterol. This is thought to stand them in good stead for the future and prevent or reduce the likelihood of later heart disease. (See chapter 4.)

Fats are split into simpler fatty substances in the gut by naturally occurring enzymes called lipases. The digestion of cows' milk fat (butterfat) by lipase leads to the release of a fatty acid, palmitic acid, which combines with calcium in the gut and is passed out in the stools, so robbing the body of calcium. In human milk, palmitic acid is built into the fat particles in such a way that when fat is digested by lipase, the acid is not released as a free fatty acid but is absorbed into the bloodstream together with part of the broken-down fat particle. In this way calcium is not lost. This is important because when babies are growing fast (and a baby grows at its fastest on the very first day of its life) they need a plentiful supply of calcium to build strong bones and teeth.

Human milk contains some lipase of its own unlike cows' milk which relies solely on lipase in the baby's intestine for its digestion. The fat in breast milk starts being digested by the milk lipase even before it reaches the gut. This means that some of the valuable fatty acids are available for use sooner than would be the case with cows' milk.

Fat is necessary for the body's development in many ways but it is especially important for the development of the outer coatings of the nerves. It seems likely that the specific pattern of fatty acids in human milk has developed in such a way as to supply the rapidly growing brain and nerves with exactly the right building materials at the right time – early infancy – when these tissues grow faster than at any other time. Clearly any disturbance in the natural balance of these essential substances may prevent optimum growth of the nerves and brain even if we cannot as yet measure the lost potential.

Less important but of more practical significance to the mother is the fact that if a breast fed baby regurgitates any milk, there is no unpleasant smell, whereas a bottle fed baby's vomit has a characteristically foul, sour smell which can quickly permeate the clothing of both mother and child. The difference is due to the presence of a fatty acid – butyric acid – in cows' milk, which smells nasty when partially digested.

Carbohydrates

Both breast milk and cows' milk contain lactose (milk sugar) but breast milk has more of it. Lactose is split into two parts in the gut – galactose and glucose – and galactose is an essential ingredient of the myelin coatings of nerve fibres. The old practice of diluting cows' milk and adding ordinary sugar (sucrose) meant that galactose was in short supply to the bottle fed baby. Some of the more recent modifications of cows' milk have included adding lactose instead of sucrose.

Breast milk also contains some glucose and some other sugars which are completely absent, or present in much lower quantities in cows' milk.

The bifidus factor is another carbohydrate present in breast milk but virtually absent from cows' milk. This is a very valuable protective factor against infection in the gut, as we'll see later in the chapter.

Minerals

Whole cows' milk (unmodified) contains almost four times as many minerals as breast milk and this is one of the reasons why a baby's kidneys have to work so hard if he is fed on cows' milk.

Modified cows' milk has much lower levels of minerals but even so there is no milk available which has the low mineral levels of breast milk. It is possible to lower the levels of the minerals in cows' milk by a process called demineralization but there is one big snag in doing this. We don't know how many useful though unknown minerals are completely removed whilst reducing the level of the ones we know exist. We just don't know the exact contents of cows' or breast milk. As these minerals are so important to the health of the baby, we'll discuss some of them in more detail.

Sodium. The level in breast milk is ideal for human babies. The level in modified cows' milk is lower than in doorstep milk but is still higher than it should be. Sodium is closely linked with water in the body and an imbalance of either can be serious and even fatal. This is why so much care must be taken of babies who are bottle fed if they develop any illness such as diarrhoea, vomiting or fever (which all reduce their water level) and why so much care must be taken not to prepare feeds which are too strong (so increasing their salt level).

Calcium, phosphorus and magnesium. Higher levels of all these are present in cows' milk, though modification reduces them to some extent. Several problems are known to have arisen from this, including a type of muscular spasm known as neonatal tetany, convulsions and poor development of the enamel of the teeth, followed by severe dental decay. For *Fluoride* see page 54.

Iron. This is one mineral present in larger amounts (twice as much) in breast milk than in unmodified cows' milk, though the levels in modified cows' milk are higher than in breast milk. Recent research indicates that the iron in breast milk is better absorbed into the bloodstream than that in cows' milk. Certain substances such as Vitamins C, E and copper help iron to be absorbed more efficiently and these are present in higher amounts in breast milk. We know that the addition of iron to milk can reduce the anti-infective properties of lactoferrin, so the low levels of iron in breast milk should not be seen as being inferior to the higher levels in modified cows' milk. The totally breast fed baby almost never becomes anaemic.

Vitamins

Breast milk contains more Vitamin A, C and E than cow's milk but less Vitamin K. In mothers well-nourished during pregnancy and having a well-balanced diet while breast feeding, there is no evidence that their fully breast fed babies need any vitamin supplements in the first six months of life. While Vitamin D supplements are unnecessary for the fully breast fed baby, the bottle fed baby needs to be given Vitamin D to prevent rickets. Most doctors still recommend that breast fed babies should have Vitamin D supplements but this stems from the earlier and incorrect assumption that breast milk contained less of the vitamin than did cows' milk. Recent research has shown that there is water soluble Vitamin D in breast milk besides the fat soluble fraction that we already knew about, and that there is more of this in human milk than in cows' milk.

The baby of a mother who is healthy and eating well will not need extra Vitamin C. Research shows that a mother's Vitamin C is concentrated in her breast milk so as to ensure that the baby gets enough. Even women who have scurvy do not produce babies deficient in Vitamin C. If the mother's diet is deficient in this vitamin, though, she'll need supplements of Vitamin C.

Now to Vitamin K. Although breast milk contains less of this vitamin than does cows' milk, there is no reason to suppose that breast fed babies should normally suffer from a lack of it. To prevent a possible shortage of Vitamin K in the newborn (which causes bleeding) many babies born in the UK are given an injection of Vitamin K after birth, whether or not the mother is going to breast feed.

Some vitamins are destroyed by heating, which is another reason why bottle fed babies can go short unless they have regular vitamin supplements.

In general, the principle should be to give any additional foods and vitamins necessary for the baby's well-being to the mother and not to the baby itself. If a mother's nutrition is good then she'll pass on all the right nutrients in her breast milk in the perfect proportions for her baby.

Anti-infective factors

We've already talked about the antibodies in breast milk but there are other substances which also help fight infection in the baby and many of these are more plentiful and more active in breast milk than in cows' milk.

The very proportion of the food substances in breast milk compared with cows' milk prevents the growth of certain organisms such as *E. coli*, dysentery and typhoid bacteria in the baby's gut. The high lactose, low phosphorus and low protein levels in particular do this.

The breast fed baby's gut, like that of the bottle fed baby, contains thousands of tiny organisms. These are of an entirely different kind in the bottle fed baby and account for the foul smell of a bottle fed baby's stools compared with the sweet smell of the stools of a breast fed baby. The organisms in the breast fed baby are members of the *Lactobacillus bifidus* family and are encouraged to grow by a special nitrogen-containing sugar – *the bifidus factor* – which is not present in useful amounts in cows' milk. The lactobacilli produce acetic and lactic acids which together prevent the growth of many disease-producing organisms such as *E. coli* (a common cause of gastro-enteritis in the bottle fed baby), the dysentery bacillus and the yeasts which cause thrush. There is also a possibility that the bifidus factor itself interferes with the 'flu virus.

An important anti-infective factor in breast milk present in much greater amounts than in cows' milk is the protein *lactoferrin*. Together with one of the immunoglobulins (IgA), lactoferrin inhibits the growth of many organisms, including *E. coli*, the yeasts and staphylococci, by robbing them of the iron they need for growth. An important discovery is that extra iron prevents this action because the organisms then have enough to use to grow and divide. So giving a breast fed baby iron supplements may actually produce more infections of the gut. To any mother whose baby has had gastro-enteritis this is far from an academic argument! Lactoferrin, like the antibodies, loses its activity when milk is boiled, so the small amount that is present in cows' milk is useless in baby milk preparations.

Three more factors interact with each other to kill bacteria: *lysozyme*, present in breast milk in an amount 300 times greater than in cows' milk; *immunoglobulin A* and a substance called *complement*. Lysozyme is present in other body secretions such as tears, where it helps prevent infections of the eyes and eyelids.

Breast milk also contains an *anti-staphylococcal factor*; *hydrogen peroxide* and *Vitamin C* which together kill bacteria such as *E. coli*; an enzyme *lactoperoxidase* which inhibits the growth of bacteria; and many *live cells*.

These live cells are white cells similar to some of those in the bloodstream. This means that breast milk is a living fluid, unlike cows' milk by the time it reaches the baby, when all the cells have been killed by processing. The lymphoid cells in breast milk make IgA as well as an anti-viral substance called *interferon*. These cells can also be absorbed from the gut into the bloodstream of the baby where they continue their work of making immunoglobulins. Other cells in breast milk are called macrophages. These are large cells which can actively engulf particles such as bacteria and also produce lactoferrin, lysozyme and complement.

Other substances which are not antibodies and yet act against certain viruses such as the polio, mumps and encephalitis viruses have been found in breast milk.

So much for the substances we *know* to be present in milk. There are undoubtedly many others that we simply haven't yet isolated, some of which may be extremely important. After all, just because something is present in large amounts or is easy to measure doesn't necessarily mean it's especially important. Perhaps some valuable parts of breast milk are as yet unknown. Various trace elements may well come into this category and it's for this reason that manufacturers of baby milks must be fighting a losing battle.

How breast milk changes

Neither breast milk nor cows' milk is of constant composition. Their make-up varies according to the length of lactation, the time of day and even within a feed itself. In the case of cows' milk these variations only affect the calf. The bottle fed baby drinks milk of highly consistent composition because cows' milk of many different types and stages is pooled for human consumption. Breast milk, on the other hand, is supplied on a 'one off' basis direct from producer to consumer and varies in composition considerably. These variations, far from being harmful, are of considerable importance as we shall now see.

Colostrum

This is the first milk made by the breast and is produced by the milk glands even before the baby is born. It is also produced for several days after birth. Colostrum is rich in protein, cells, minerals, Vitamins A, E and B_{12} and has less fat and sugar than later milk. By the time a breast fed baby is one week old it has five times the Vitamin E that a bottle fed baby has in its body. A difference readily apparent to the mother is that her very first milk looks 'yellower' than the milk that follows. Most important, though, is the fact that the protein fraction of colostrum contains large amounts of antibodies – the same ones that are present in later milk but many more of them. These give the newborn baby resistance to infection at a time when he would otherwise be particularly susceptible. The antibodies also coat the gut lining, which not only prevents organisms from entering the bloodstream but also blocks the absorption of proteins which might set up allergic responses.

Bottle fed babies in the Western world don't even get cows' colostrum, let alone human colostrum, yet dairy cows' colostrum (or beestings) is considered so vital for calves that farmers save it for them or even go to the expense of buying it if necessary.

Colostrum looks thick and yellow and often leaks from the nipples during the second half of pregnancy. By the third day after birth it becomes more milky and is sometimes called 'transitional milk' but there is no sudden change from one to the other. There is not a fixed amount of colostrum, as many people think, so expressing it ante-natally will not reduce the total supply available to the baby. Letting the baby suck frequently for as long as he wants in the first few days will not only give him more of this valuable colostrum but will also hasten the production of mature milk and will condition the let-down reflex to work quickly and efficiently. (See page 22.)

The low fat content of colostrum is advantageous to the newborn baby because he secretes little lipase of his own and would have difficulty in digesting larger amounts of fat in the first day or so.

An anti-trypsin factor in colostrum (also present in mature milk) helps prevent the digestion of antibodies by trypsin in the gut. Antibodies, as we've seen, are proteins and the gut's trypsin breaks down proteins under normal circumstances. To ensure that these life-saving antibodies are not destroyed, colostrum contains this special anti-trypsin enzyme.

Mature milk

This contains a fifth of the protein of colostrum and more fat and sugar. It is thinner-looking and whiter or even bluish-white. During the first year of breast feeding the protein content of breast milk gradually falls, regardless of the mother's diet. This is compensated for by the fact that most babies are given increasing amounts of solid foods from about six months and these provide the extra protein necessary for growth. Also, don't forget that the baby is growing at its fastest in the first six months of life when the level of protein in breast milk is at its highest. The fall off in protein is paralleled by this normal reduction in growth rate.

As we saw in the last chapter, the early part of a feed is made up of the foremilk which is low in fat while the later part is the hindmilk with four to five times the amount of fat and one-and-a-half times as much protein. Some mixing occurs when a feed begins. This happens more in the second breast. Many hungry babies whose mothers think they are not producing enough milk are only getting the low calorie foremilk before the mother stops feeding. As a result the baby actually loses weight or fails to gain and is soon started on cows' milk supplements.

The reason for this problem is that the mother's let-down reflex may be poorly conditioned so the hindmilk is only let down late in a feed. As foremilk constitutes only about a third of the available milk in each breast, the baby gradually starves. The important thing to be learned from this is that frequent feeds in the early days condition the let-down reflex to work well and so supply all the milk a baby could want.

The changing composition of milk during a feed may help a baby develop his own appetite control mechanism. A baby finishes feeding at the first breast with high fat milk and then slakes his thirst at the second breast with the thin, watery foremilk. Babies have been seen to stop feeding at the first breast even though there is still milk there. They then go on to feed with vigour at the second breast, much to everyone's surprise. Similarly, babies often stop feeding at the second breast of their own accord even though there is plenty of milk there. This may well be because the baby has had enough of the fat rich hindmilk. This early development of appetite control could well be a factor in the prevention of obesity later in life. A baby has to learn to control his appetite and this is very difficult to do if he is given cows' milk of constant composition. A bottle fed baby drinks large volumes to quench his thirst and in so doing takes in too many calories. Soon he's fat and we now know that many fat babies tend to become fat adults.

Regression milk

When lactation ends, the milk becomes more like colostrum – thicker and yellower. Some women find they are able to express this milk from their breasts many months after they have stopped feeding their babies.

So now we've examined the complexity and specificity of breast milk, is it fair to assume that bottle fed babies really do so badly? The answer is that while the vast majority of bottle fed babies to thrive, more of them suffer from illness during their first year and there may be many long-term effects of drinking cows' milk in infancy which we are only now beginning to appreciate. We'll discuss this more in chapter 4. The basic thing we've tried to get across in this chapter is that breast milk *is* different from cows' milk, even if the cows' milk is modified. It's no longer reasonable for doctors and food scientists to tell the public that breast milk is unnecessary – today we know better.

Having said this, there will still be mothers who decide not to breast feed even though they know that breast milk is best, so we must be thankful that there is an alternative to breast milk. In other countries, especially in the third world, it might have been better for babies had cows' milk never been available as a substitute. The vast majority of babies in these areas would have fared much better on breast milk. Bottle feeding, however carefully done, can only ever be a second best. Nature gives a mother the very best for her baby.

4 Best for baby?

When weighing up the pros and cons of breast feeding, the scale falls very heavily on the side of the 'pros' and indeed when writing this and the next chapter we found it difficult to find anything much to say against breast feeding. Even many of the 'disadvantages' that would-be breast feeders see are easily overcome if you know how.

Benefits to the baby

There is an increasing body of scientific evidence to support the medical advantages enjoyed by breast fed babies. The first reports that breast fed babies might be healthier came early this century, soon after the mass introduction of bottle feeding. A trickle of information continued over the years and has developed into an avalanche in the last five years or so. The medical and nursing professions are not always quick to take up new information, especially if it recommends sweeping changes in the management of people in hospital and the community. This is not necessarily a bad thing and does protect the public from medical fads and fancies to some extent. But in the case of breast feeding we think that if *mothers* understand the advantages to their babies of being breast fed, then pressure from them will do more than anything to change the poor standard of help and advice available to most breast feeding women in this country.

The perfect food

In the last chapter we explained the unique composition of breast milk and how the amount and type of each foodstuff is just right for your baby. But breast milk doesn't simply provide food, as we shall now see.

Perfect for growth

A myth has grown up in the Western world that healthy babies are fat babies. This has meant that women have fed their babies in such a way as to make them as 'bonny' as possible as quickly as possible. It is an undeniable fact that bottle fed babies double their birth weight quicker than most breast feds and that this produces more obesity in infancy and later life (see page 52).

But growing isn't only a matter of getting fatter quicker, as many people think. The growth of the human infant is a complex affair. When we compare the rates of growth of infants in the developing countries with those in ours we find that their 'underprivileged' children grow less quickly than ours in the West. As prosperity increases so do the growth rates of babies. But is it sensible to assume that babies that grow fast are what we should be aiming for?

Apparently not, if the work of a distinguished doctor in southern Africa is anything to go by. He questions whether the usual growth rate for American and British babies should be taken as normal. By their standards many millions of children are malnourished yet seem perfectly fit and well and grow up to be healthier than many Western children. A hundred years ago English children reached their maximum height at the age of 25 – today they get there at 16. Among the rural Bantu in Africa today the age is 20.

Animal experiments have shown that slower growth rates in the young make for slow ageing and this seems to be borne out in humans if we accept evidence from South Africa where in one study there were at least twenty times as many Bantu over the age of 100 than there were whites. This is well worth thinking about because it may be that by force feeding our children we could be accelerating their growth and the onset of degenerative diseases, so decreasing their life span. It's almost impossible to overfeed grossly if you're only breast feeding yet it's the easiest thing in the world if you're using cows' milk to which you can also add cereals and other solids. There is every reason to suppose that the amounts of nutrients in breast milk are perfectly geared to the optimum rate of growth of the child (especially to the human baby's fast brain growth rate). Any tampering with this can produce problems.

Fewer infections

We saw in the last chapter that breast milk contains many factors that protect a baby from infection by bacteria, viruses, yeasts and other organisms. This sounds good but in practical terms how important is it today when hygienic precautions for bottle feeding are so good and the treatment of infections so advanced?

For two thirds of the world's population, feeding babies with cows' milk is 'tantamount to signing a death warrant', according to the United Nations Protein Advisory Group. The risk of these babies developing infective diarrhoea is extremely high, because of the lack of adequate hygienic precautions together with the lack of anti-infective factors in the cows' milk. In the Western world we don't have the mortality figures that we had in the earlier part of this century but we do still have many thousands of babies suffering from gastro-enteritis and respiratory infections (colds, coughs, croup, ear infections, pneumonia, bronchiolitis and 'flu, to name but a few). Some of our babies also get more serious infections such as meningitis and septicaemia. Though we can prevent most of these babies from actually dying, no mother wants to see her baby in hospital or even suffering from repeated infections at home. *Breast feeding will help protect your baby against these infections, especially if you breast feed exclusively*. It is now almost certain that even one feed of bottle milk can so alter the baby's bowel (albeit temporarily) that he can pick up an infection that a wholely breast fed baby would not.

In Manchester in 1970, out of 170 babies under six months old admitted to a hospital with gastro-enteritis, *only one* baby was being breast fed!

In Newcastle in 1976, among babies treated for respiratory infections, only one baby in fourteen was being breast fed, compared with one in four among healthy babies outside the hospital.

If we look further afield, we can find even more startling

figures. In parts of rural Chile in 1973, bottle fed babies had twice the chance of dying as had breast fed babies. In Guatemala in 1971, experienced workers reported that gastro-enteritis was unknown in the breast fed but common in bottle fed babies. And in Canadian Eskimos in 1971, middle ear infections were five times as common in the bottle fed!

We know that today the vast majority of western mothers prepare feeds hygienically. So it must be that the many anti-infective factors in breast milk are responsible in a *positive* way for the resistance of the breast fed to infection.

Two rare diseases of babies that we'll mention here are necrotising enterocolitis – a bowel infection with a high death rate seen almost exclusively in the bottle fed – and acrodermatitis enteropathica, a disease of unknown cause for which breast milk provides the only treatment. These are rare diseases but virtually never seen in the breast fed child.

Fewer allergic diseases

There are probably few subjects in child care that have stimulated so much interest and concern in recent years as has infantile eczema and it continues to be a distressing and difficult condition to treat. An American study that followed over 20,000 babies for five years found that there were seven times as many babies with eczema in the bottle fed group as in those completely breast fed. (Babies given some breast and some bottle milk were twice as likely to get eczema as the totally breast fed ones.) This survey also found that one in twenty babies fed on cows' milk developed eczema!

In fact, more than 30,000 babies develop cows' milk allergy every year in the USA and there must be many more that simply aren't diagnosed.

This research into allergy is fascinating. It has been known for some time that eczema, asthma and hay fever are less common in children who have been breast fed. We now know that many other illnesses are caused by allergy to cows' milk protein or to other food proteins that pass through the gut wall of bottle fed babies.

As we mentioned in the last chapter, babies only begin to make their own immunoglobulin A (IgA) after the first few weeks of life. Until they make enough, they need IgA from their mothers' milk. Cows' milk IgA is no help as it is spoilt by heat treatment. IgA is important in preventing allergic diseases because it forms a protective coating over the gut lining and not only fights infection there but also stops large protein molecules (such as infective organisms or proteins from cows' milk or solid foods) leaking through the gut wall into the bloodstream.

In babies who are bottle fed there is no protective coating of IgA until the baby makes enough of its own (probably not for three months or so). Thus food proteins can leak into the bloodstream through the gut wall and be taken to various parts of the body where, in susceptible people, they set up an allergic response. This allergy may not produce symptoms straight away but may take a while to show itself. *Unfortunately a single bottle of cows' milk can sensitize a baby and so possibly cause allergic symptoms either at once, when he next takes cows' milk or some time later*. The only way of proving whether symptoms are caused by an allergy or not is to remove what is thought to be the offending food from the baby's diet, wait for the symptoms to disappear, then reintroduce the food and see whether the same symptoms recur. This has been done with cows' milk protein allergy and the case proved many times over.

Why haven't we heard about this before, we can hear you say, and does cows' milk allergy cause any other problems?

Until recently, the diagnosis of cows' milk allergy or allergy to any other food was not clinically respectable and medical students were scarcely taught about it. Various studies have suggested that between about ½ per cent and 7 per cent of bottle fed babies are affected by an allergy to cows' milk. Symptoms produced vary tremendously and include diarrhoea, vomiting, failure to thrive, bleeding from the gut with consequent anaemia, colic, eczema, nettle rash, runny nose, cough, wheezing and rattling of the chest, asthma and bronchiolitis.

The food protein most commonly involved is the β-lactoglobulin in cows' milk. There is no β-lactoglobulin in breast milk. Boys seem to be affected twice as often as girls and the symptoms seem to be more common in families with a tendency to allergic problems. Obviously a baby does not have all the various symptoms at once and they may come and go with spontaneous remissions between attacks. The child who always seems to have a cold may in fact be allergic to some particular foodstuff and the 'cold' may be an allergic condition of the lining of the nose and not a viral infection at all.

In a study looking at eczema in children it has been found that among children from 'allergic' families, 50 per cent develop eczema in infancy if they are bottle fed whereas only 8 per cent get it if they are breast fed. As breast feeding obviously gives such protection against eczema in these circumstances and as eczema can be such an unpleasant complaint, this argument alone is a strong point in favour of breast feeding.

In a study in Lancashire 90 per cent of mothers with an allergic family history were able to breast feed in hospital and 80 per cent were still feeding at three months. This remarkably high level of success was due to two factors. First, the doctors were very encouraging and the women had plenty of back-up help, and second, they were highly motivated because they were so convinced of the value of breast feeding to their potentially allergic children.

It is possible for breast milk to contain traces of 'foreign' food proteins (such as egg, cows' milk, cereal, nut and fish proteins) which can cause allergic symptoms in highly susceptible babies. This helps explain why a few breast fed babies develop eczema and asthma. Mothers of susceptible babies should as far as possible avoid eating large amounts of these protein foods at any one time. Other ways a breast fed baby can get eczema and asthma are by the inhalation of or skin contact with 'foreign' proteins.

Less coeliac disease

Coeliac disease is a condition seen in children after they begin to eat cereals and is caused by the gut's inability to handle the protein *gluten* which is present in wheat, rye, barley and oats. The gut lining is damaged by this protein so that the digestion of various foods is impaired. Such children fail to thrive and have a swollen abdomen and foul-smelling stools. Treatment consists of completely withdrawing gluten from the diet. A recent government report on infant feeding advised that babies should not be given cereals (or indeed any solids) before about four months in order to protect young babies from the possibility of getting coeliac disease.

It seems likely that the IgA coating of the gut lining in young breast fed babies may prevent this damage by gluten. In any case it seems wise not to give cereals at least until the baby is making enough of his own IgA after the first four months or so.

In a survey in Western Ireland where only 3 per cent of babies are breast fed, coeliac disease is about four times as common as in England where many more babies are breast fed.

Less ulcerative colitis and Crohn's disease

These two diseases of later life may be connected with the type of feeding in infancy and especially the early introduction of solids. In one survey it was found that people with ulcerative colitis were twice as likely as 'normal' people never to have been breast fed.

Another study showed that people with longstanding ulcerative colitis had high levels of antibodies to cows' milk protein in their blood.

More research into this aspect of these diseases is obviously needed. The difficulty with this sort of research, though, is that few adults know exactly how they themselves were fed as babies, so the researchers need to ask the subjects' mothers for details which is a very time-consuming business.

Fewer cot deaths

These are sudden deaths of babies (usually under six months old) for which no obvious cause is found at post mortem. A viral illness is suggested in many cases. The babies go to sleep quite normally and then die in their sleep. In this country two in every 1,000 babies die in this way – a total of 1,800 babies a year! It is not difficult to imagine the immense suffering caused to the parents of these children.

Research into cot deaths is rather confused as many workers talk only about the method of feeding during the first few weeks of life and not that at the time of death. What does emerge, though, is that the risk to a breast fed baby is very much less than that to a bottle fed baby. Even if breast feeding is only done for a short time some protection is conferred against the risk of cot death later. There have been isolated cases of entirely breast fed babies dying but these seem to be rare.

No one knows why these babies die but some researchers have suggested that there might be a sudden overwhelming allergic response to a 'foreign' protein such as cows' milk protein. Another idea is that the baby is killed by a viral invasion with which he is completely unable to cope. Because breast milk contains no 'foreign' protein and also provides resistance against many viral infections, these facts alone suggest that a good way of preventing many of these tragic deaths would be for all babies to be completely breast fed for *at least* the first four months.

Less obesity

It is an interesting observation that the babies winning baby competitions twenty years ago were all 'bonny' babies – fat and podgy – whereas today a baby like this wouldn't get a second glance from the judges. We've become very weight conscious, especially over the last decade or so, partly because we know that besides looking unattractive, fat people are more prone to heart disease, high blood pressure, diabetes, varicose veins and gallstones and also have a reduced life expectancy.

The statement that fat babies become fat adults is an oversimplification and in many cases is not true. However, there is certainly an overall tendency for this to happen, especially if the rate of weight gain in early infancy is high and it has been shown that 80 per cent of fat babies become fat adults. What is certain is that the habit of eating too much is easily implanted in a young child. While we have all seen fat breast fed babies, there is statistically much more chance of a baby being fat if bottle fed, as many surveys have shown. In one such study in Sheffield in 1971, 60 per cent of bottle fed babies put on too much weight in the first year compared with only 19 per cent of breast fed babies.

One of the reasons for this is that the high mineral content of cows' milk makes babies thirsty and if their thirst is quenched by more milk, the extra calories make them fat. The recent modification of cows' milk preparations, which means their mineral content is better controlled, may reduce this danger to some extent. However, some mothers will always give their babies 'an extra scoop for the pot', especially before bedtime and this just can't happen when a baby is breast fed. Another reason is that it's easy to put some cereal powder into a bottle in an attempt to make the baby sleep longer. Breast feeding mothers are much less likely to give their babies early solids.

Less heart disease

Many people are amazed at the suggestion that heart disease could possibly have anything to do with baby milk. Several research reports must make them think again.

A study of a hundred bodies of young people aged between 0 and 20 who had died from various unrelated causes showed that abnormalities in the coronary arteries were more common in those who had been bottle fed. Abnormality in the coronary arteries is the major problem underlying angina and heart attacks so is clearly worth worrying about. One in three men in the Western world dies of heart disease.

There are several theories as to why this should be. Some have suggested that the arterial damage in the bottle fed is a result of the action of antibodies to cows' milk protein which are found in bottle fed babies. Others think that the different fat composition and content of cows' milk may be responsible.

The discovery that men under 60 who have heart attacks have higher than normal levels of antibodies to cows' milk protein made a lot of people sit up and rethink their ideas. It has also been found that a man who has had a heart attack has three times more chance of dying from it if he has any cows' milk antibodies in his blood at all.

Although breast fed babies *can* develop antibodies to cows' milk later in life, there is evidence that when they do their antibody levels are lower than those of people who were fed on cows' milk as infants.

Cows' milk protein causes the formation of antibodies in susceptible people when they drink it. These antibodies or 'immune complexes' are known to make the blood more sticky and so predispose towards clot formation. The ability to produce antibodies to cows' milk protein may well be inherited; one family in which there was a very high level of heart disease had antibody levels eight times those seen in the normal population.

Although the research is not as yet conclusive, it seems likely that some bottle fed babies become sensitized by cows' milk protein, develop antibodies to it and so become more likely to suffer from heart attacks in later life. Even if this theory offers only a glimmer of hope, the fact remains that degenerative arterial disease is a forerunner of angina and heart attacks – diseases so serious and common in the Western world that any suggestion of a causative factor should be taken very seriously.

It's important, though, to stress that we're not suggesting that breast feeding will completely prevent heart attacks. Heart disease is so complex and the numbers of factors involved so many that even though bottle feeding is probably one of the factors, it certainly isn't the only one.

Less dental decay

The breast fed baby is less likely to suffer from dental decay when he is older than the bottle fed baby, a fact which is little known. Dental decay not only costs the National Health Service a lot of money (only mental disease costs more) but, more important, it causes children a lot of pain and brings with it the risk of having to have false teeth. Just bear in mind that 37 per cent of all the people in the UK over the age of 16 have no teeth of their own and you'll see how serious the problem is. There are 22 million people who actually have false teeth and we have seen four-year-olds with complete sets of dentures!

So why is the breast fed baby protected? We don't know for certain but there seem to be two mechanisms at work. Firstly, the fluoride level in breast milk is increased in areas with high levels of fluoride in the drinking water. It seems that cows' milk produced in fluoridated water areas doesn't show as great an increase, though the fluoride content of the milk does rise slightly compared with that from non-fluoridated areas. We know that fluoride in the right dose reduces dental decay by 50 per cent so this is one protective factor.

However, in a non-fluoridated area, the amount of fluoride in breast and bottle milk is nearly the same but breast fed babies still have reduced decay rates in early childhood. This means that another mechanism must be at work. In one survey it was shown that children breast fed for more than three months in an area with little fluoride in the water had a 46 per cent reduction in the incidence of dental decay compared with bottle fed children. In practical terms this meant that the numbers of decayed, missing or filled teeth were almost twice as high in those children who had been bottle fed!

Before you jump up and say that this was obviously because of the sugar added to the babies' bottles, the research workers thought of that and managed to show that sugar was not involved in the differences seen.

The same sort of study in a different area with fluoridated water showed that children breast fed for more than three months had a 50 per cent reduction in the incidence of dental decay compared with the bottle fed.

Better jaw and mouth development

Many specialists report that they see fewer problems with faulty jaw and mouth development in breast fed babies. Indeed, in one survey of nearly 500 children with such problems only two had been breast fed. The underlying cause seems to be the abnormal swallowing mechanism that a bottle fed baby learns when sucking from the bottle teat.

This abnormal 'swallow' can produce several types of malocculusion of the teeth, all of which take much time and patience on the part of the orthodontist, child and parents to put right. Treatment for many of these disorders often means repeated trips to the dentist over a period of years – well worth preventing if possible.

Multiple sclerosis
Some researchers have suggested a possible connection between bottle feeding and the later development of multiple sclerosis. Further work is in progress at present.

Other developmental differences
Whilst it is relatively unimportant, it is interesting that two studies have shown that breast fed babies *walk* earlier than bottle fed babies even after allowing for differences in weight between the two groups and excluding babies whose mothers went out to work (because they might possibly have been less stimulated to walk).

Another study of nearly 400 children using several tests showed that the highest *intelligence quotients* were obtained by children who had been breast fed for between four and nine months. Five per cent of the breast fed children had IQs of 130 or higher, while none of the bottle fed group had. Before dismissing this survey as being a lot of nonsense, it is worth considering that it's likely that the amino acid pattern of human milk is optimal for the development of the human brain, which grows tremendously fast in the first year of life.

Attachment to mother
Scientific proof of any increased attachment to the mother if her child is breast fed is hard to come by but a closer relationship seems likely if only because the baby has to depend on his mother alone for food. She is also likely to feed him to comfort him instead of just holding him or giving him a dummy. Studies have in fact shown that breast fed babies spend less time in their cots and more with their mothers than bottle fed ones. In communities where unrestricted breast feeding is not only allowed but is actively encouraged by society, mothers don't let their babies cry even for a short time. In our Western society babies are often left to cry in their cots because 'it's not time for a feed' and 'they might be spoilt if they're picked up for a cuddle'. The baby whose mother gives him the breast for food or comfort whenever he cries would seem highly likely to grow up more secure in his mother's love.

Studies have shown that the behaviour of a breast feeding mother before, during and after feeding is also different from that of a bottle feeding mother. The mother who breast feeds is more likely to kiss, rock and touch her baby while the bottle feeding mother is more likely to rub, pat and jiggle her baby and will also show much more concern over 'wind'.

The properly breast fed baby, cries from hunger less because his needs can be immediately satisfied by warm milk. The bottle fed baby is more likely to have to wait until his mother thinks it is time for his feed and then will have to wait again while his feed is prepared and warmed and may feel very real hunger and frustration during this time. What's more, the breast fed baby can be sure of a decent meal, even in countries where his mother is relatively short of food herself, while the bottle fed baby in a poor family may be given a dilute feed which won't satisfy him for long. This is, unfortunately, especially likely in the third world.

So much for all the advantages of breast feeding for your baby. Quite a list, isn't it? We often hear advocates of bottle feeding say 'Yes, but look at the millions of babies who have grown up healthily on cows' milk.' Our answer is that breast fed babies not only grow up *even more* healthily but also that breast feeding *can actually save lives.* We already know of many diseases linked with bottle feeding and who knows how many more will be discovered in the future?

Are there any disadvantages to breast feeding from the baby's point of view? Only a few, which can be overcome.

If a mother's diet is *grossly* deficient in protein and fat (such as may happen among the starving peoples of the world) then the baby is liable to go short as well. The answer here is not to give the baby cows' milk but to give the mother more food. The World Health Organization recently decided that in future it would concentrate famine relief monies on food for breast feeding mothers rather than on vast and costly supplies of powdered cows' milk. Babies fed on cows' milk in famine circumstances have a much greater risk of dying than do breast fed babies, because of the enormous risk of gastro-enteritis from unsterilized bottles and water. They are also highly likely to be given dilute feeds so that the mother can save her supplies of milk powder in case she can't get any or can't afford any the next day.

Another problem crops up in countries where mothers eat large amounts of polished rice which is lacking in Vitamin B_1 (thiamine) and develop beri-beri. Breast fed babies can become acutely ill when fed by these mothers. The solution is for health workers to teach mothers where they are going wrong – the rice should be eaten unpolished in order to provide enough Vitamin B_1.

Some vegetarian mothers have low levels of Vitamin B_{12} in their milk and so give too little of this vitamin to their babies, which then develop symptoms of deficiency.

And in this country? The only serious disadvantage is probably the frustration and hunger suffered by a baby whose mother has inadequate milk for him. But this is almost always easily overcome with help and perseverance (see chapter 10).

5 Best for you?

Advantages to you

Satisfaction

The mother who breast feeds her baby successfully for as long as she and the baby both want is likely to get a lot of satisfaction from doing the right thing for her baby, even if she doesn't know of all the very real physical advantages to him. Many mothers say that they felt a tremendous sense of loss when they gave their baby its last breast feed. Perhaps this is partly because a breast fed baby is even more dependent upon its mother for its food than is a bottle fed one, and the majority of mothers enjoy this feeling of being needed. Whilst on the subject of satisfaction it is interesting that in a survey of recently delivered mothers, those who were 'greatly pleased' with their babies were much more successful at breast feeding than those who were 'indifferent'.

Fulfilment

Another feeling often expressed is that breast feeding is one of the things that only a woman can do – like giving birth. In today's world of sexual equality and unisex this feminine fulfilment is valued not only by the naturally maternal but also by the erstwhile career woman who sees the enjoyment of breast feeding as representing the female part of her character. This oneness that many breast feeding women feel with their babies is often quoted as the major advantage to breast feeding mothers. Certainly they often seem to be more at ease with their babies. One survey showed that breast feeding mothers were three times as likely to sleep with their babies as were bottle feeders.

Getting your figure back

Three months after your baby is born you're more likely to be losing weight without dieting than the mother who is bottle feeding. Breast feeding uses up some of the fat stores accumulated during pregnancy and so naturally helps you get back to your pre-pregnancy shape and weight. If the shape of your breasts is altered at all, it will probably be because of the pregnancy and not the breast feeding. Breasts tend to return to their normal shape and size about six months after weaning. Various women report that their breasts are either smaller, larger or droopier after breast feeding but there is no general trend.

Convenience

A big practical point in favour of breast feeding is that it really is more convenient. More convenient not only at home, where there are no bottles and teats to wash and sterilize and no feeds to prepare but also when you go out as there is no equipment to get ready and take with you. Holidays become a much more practical proposition and car rides with the baby can actually be pleasant. Not for you the cooling of a bottle of hot milk by holding it out of the car window at great speed! And no spilt milk powder over the car seats.

The breast feeding mother needs only her baby and a clean nappy to go anywhere and it takes only a little ingenuity and forethought to be able to breast feed anywhere without embarrassment to you or anyone else.

Another thing that only a mother who has both breast and bottle fed at different times will know is that it's nearly always possible to comfort an infant by giving him the breast, even if he's not particularly hungry. Bottle fed babies often don't seem to be comforted by sucking on a bottle of water or a dummy – unless you're lucky. This means that a household with a breast fed baby is quieter and happier all round than one with a bottle fed baby, provided you as his mother are willing to let him be comforted by suckling him whenever he cries.

Cost

The question of the relative cost of bottle feeding as against breast feeding is not really of very great importance in Western countries. Few people are literally on the bread line and a few pence here or there will not influence the average woman either way.

The cost of dried milk powder needs to be added to the cost of bottles, teats, sterilizing tablets or gas or electricity to boil the equipment, when working out the cost of bottle feeding. A bottle feeding mother will need several bottles and teats over the total period and the cost of these soon adds up.

A breast feeding mother needs to consider the cost of the extra food she should be eating each day in order to produce enough milk. Experts think that she needs to eat enough extra food to provide her with 300–500 calories a day over and above her normal intake. The baby will take more from her than this amount but the difference is made up by the calories obtained from the fat stores she laid down during pregnancy. This is why a breast feeding mother will carry on losing weight (unless she eats too much) until she stops breast feeding.

Obviously the cost of extra food will depend entirely on what sort of food the breast feeding mother chooses to eat – if she takes her extra calories as rump steak and avocado pear it'll work out far more expensive than if she takes them as a glass of milk and cheese sandwiches. If she just eats a little more of everything than she normally eats, then the cost of the extra food is lower than the cost of bottle feeding a baby. This is especially important in the underdeveloped countries where many mothers literally cannot afford to buy cows' milk but can just about afford to buy some extra food for themselves.

Birth control

The contraceptive effect of breast feeding was dismissed as an old wives' tale until very recently. This is doubly amazing as it is the only contraceptive known to the majority of the world's women. It is quite true that a woman is less likely to conceive while breast feeding even if she uses no other form of contraception but what is not so often realized is that it *is* possible for her to conceive while still breast feeding. The amount of protection depends upon whether the baby relies solely on breast milk, on the length of time between feeds, and on whether the baby is allowed to feed for comfort after or between feeds.

Why should conception be less likely? The answer seems to be that the high levels of the hormone prolactin in the breast feeding mother inhibit the response of her ovaries to the pituitary gland's follicle-stimulating hormone. Ovulation therefore doesn't occur and pregnancy can't happen.

However, prolactin levels naturally fall throughout lactation, even in a fully breast feeding mother, so there comes a time when they are no longer high enough to prevent ovulation. In *fully* breast feeding women this doesn't happen until around the tenth week at the *very* earliest and even then *only one woman in twenty* will ovulate before the eighteenth week after childbirth. The average length of time before the return of periods in a mother who is fully breast feeding for six to eight months and then giving the breast for drinks and comfort when the baby starts on solids, is over fourteen months!

In women who don't breast feed at all, ovulation occurs *on average* eight to ten weeks after the birth of their babies; this means that one in two will be at risk of becoming pregnant before her baby is eight to ten weeks old unless she uses some other form of contraception.

The partially breast feeding mother will not ovulate for longer than the average bottle feeding mother but for less time than the fully breast feeding mother.

It is not safe to wait for your first period before you start using contraception because 5 per cent of women ovulate before their first period. Usually, though, the first few menstrual cycles after childbirth are anovular.

Many studies in far-flung parts of the world suggest that the birth controlling effect of full breast feeding is in fact more powerful there than in the Western world. (The interval between babies is around two to three years for many women in underdeveloped countries.) Breast feeding mothers in these countries are often undernourished and this can cause a delay in ovulation. In some cases there are tribal taboos on sexual intercourse with lactating women. Also, many of these women are far more likely than we are to practise completely unrestricted breast feeding. The sort of complete breast feeding most often seen in the Western world is based on the baby having five or six feeds a day (which is really only token breast feeding) whereas babies in the rest of the world are fed many more times than this. When there are long periods between suckling, which there are with only five or six feeds a day, the high prolactin levels in the blood aren't kept up. It is thought that the low levels of prolactin occurring in these long intervals between feeds allow ovulation to occur. Similarly, when the baby is given solids or supplementary bottle feeds he'll gradually rely less and less on breast milk for his nourishment and the decreased suckling will quickly lower prolactin levels and allow ovulation to occur.

It seems sensible, therefore, for the Western woman not to rely on breast feeding as a method of contraception, even if she feeds frequently, though she need not worry about using any other method for the first ten weeks if she's *fully breast feeding* her baby in the natural way. In contrast, the bottle feeding mother is well advised to use some form of birth control as soon as she starts having intercourse again.

Breast cancer

It has long been thought that breast feeding protects a woman from the eventual likelihood of getting cancer of the breast. It is a fact that in those areas of the world where women spend many years of their lives breast feeding, breast cancer is very rare indeed. But this doesn't necessarily mean that it's the breast feeding that's protecting them and there's no evidence that such a mechanism works in Western women with their 'token' breast feeding. We still don't know what does cause this cancer – the commonest cancer of women. There's certainly *no* evidence that breast feeding is a contributory cause of breast cancer.

Some possible disadvantages of breast feeding

If there are so many good reasons why breast feeding is better for mothers, why do so many women decide not to do it at all? It would be foolish to pretend that there were no drawbacks – but they're mostly easily overcome, as we'll see.

You'll be unfashionable

Probably the biggest disadvantage most women see is that breast feeding is unfashionable. In maternity wards it has often been noticed by the staff that if one mother is breast feeding successfully, newly delivered mothers are likely to copy her. If she fails, though, other mothers are likely to stop breast feeding too!

When bottle feeding first became 'fashionable' only the relatively wealthy could afford to buy milk powder and bottles but gradually the habit spread through all the social groups until today, when low-earning families are those most likely to contain a bottle fed baby. The fashion is now changing back again and once more the middle classes are leading the way.

You'll feel un-sexy

The next great disadvantage many women imagine is that breast feeding will make them less sexy in their own eyes and in those of their husbands. The cult of the breast as a sex object has undoubtedly helped speed the decline of breast feeding. The up-pointed, conical breast of the fifties and sixties seemed to be there solely to attract men. Certainly very few babies ever got a look in! Perhaps the recent trend towards more natural living with many young women doing without bras and make-up and relying more on their inborn femininity to attract men will also release their breasts to perform their more natural function.

You'll feel immodest

Breasts in our society have become equated with sex and women who choose to breast feed and thus reveal their breasts are thought by many to be immodest. At the beginning of the century no one turned a hair at the sight of a woman feeding her baby in public. Now breast feeding must be done with more than a passing thought for modesty or else the mother runs the risk of people turning to stare. This fear of embarrassment is a great off-putter to many women who may be embarrassed not only at the thought of feeding in front of complete strangers but also in front of relatives – even their husbands and children.

The swing back to breast feeding in the early seventies started with the better educated, freer thinking mothers who realized that feeding their babies offered advantages both to them and to their babies which far outweighed any feelings of embarrassment they might have had. As more and more women breast feed, feeding in public is becoming gradually more acceptable. But until TV and other areas of the media start showing mothers feeding, the move towards acceptability will be slow.

You'll feel disgusted

Allied to this feeling of embarrassment is a very real feeling of disgust at the idea of breast feeding. Mothers who feel this way refuse to breast feed at all or else give up after a day or two because to them it seems too animal-like. It's unlikely that anything will make them change their minds but one good way to help stop girls from growing up with these deep-rooted feelings is to introduce lessons mentioning breast feeding along with other aspects of child rearing at school. Some education authorities already encourage such lessons as part of the school curriculum and in mixed schools there is the added advantage that boys can discuss the subject too. In one area of London, local health educators take a nursing mother with them to these classes. Until children grow up in an environment where breast feeding is commonplace and 'normal' there is bound to be some sense of disgust in society as a whole.

It'll hurt

Many women who have never breast fed imagine that it'll be painful and so never try.

It is true that many women who breast feed do have sore nipples and a few have other painful breast conditions. Painful nipples are only temporary and the majority of the other painful conditions are mostly avoidable. In a study in Blackburn nearly one woman in six who stopped breast feeding did so because her nipples were sore. We now know that they stopped unnecessarily – their nipple soreness would have gone spontaneously if they had carried on feeding.

You'll be tied

A more practical drawback to breast feeding in our society is that it can be inconvenient because it ties the mother to her child. If she is to breast feed successfully and fully for at least four to six months, then she'll need to be with her baby almost constantly during that time. There are ways round this, though. Some mothers learn the knack of expressing enough milk into a bottle for someone else to give the baby while they go out and others give their babies the occasional bottle of cows' milk. We don't like the latter method because until about four months the baby is still vulnerable to the effects of cows' milk protein and so shouldn't have it at all.

Certainly in the first few weeks, outings without the baby will have to be limited because the baby won't go long between feeds. Even a trip to the supermarket with Dad babysitting can be tricky but there are ways round this (see chapters 9 and 14).

You can't see how much he's getting

We live in a society that measures everything, and anything that can't be measured is often regarded with suspicion. A midwife once asked us why Nature didn't provide women with transparent breasts. Our answer was, why didn't bottle manufacturers make bottles in opaque material – it wouldn't have discouraged breast feeding mothers so much.

We've been brainwashed into thinking that it's important to know exactly how much milk the baby has taken but of course it very rarely is important, especially if the baby is healthy and thriving – which he will be if breast feeding is properly managed. No two babies are alike and so each baby will want different amounts at different times of the day. Properly managed breast feeding is a perfectly balanced supply and demand system.

You'll have to feed more often

Breast fed babies do need more frequent feeding than bottle fed babies and many mothers find that the feeds take longer until their let-down reflex is working well. For a busy mother with several children this can mean that other jobs such as meticulous housework have to be sacrificed.

Unless a mother is warned in advance, she may resent the fact that her breast fed baby needs feeding perhaps two or three times a night, whereas her friends' bottle fed babies go through the night at an early age. The answer here is to organize things so that night feeds interfere with sleep as little as possible rather than deciding not to breast feed. (See chapter 8.)

You might fail

We're convinced that the biggest disadvantage that breast feeding has in the Western world is that the mother fears she'll fail and, as a result, often does. This can produce long-lasting psychological effects including a very deep sense of disappointment. So great can this feeling of failure be that many doctors and nurses have refused to tell mothers just how important it is to feed their babies themselves, for fear of their being unable to do so. This is a tragic situation not only because many mothers and babies are now not even trying but also because babies are being done out of their natural food and mothers out of their natural right – all for nothing.

The situation for many mothers today is that they feed their babies ten minutes a side every four hours or so during the day and once or not at all at night, because that is what the hospital told them to do. With this 'token' breast feeding they find that their milk supplies are dwindling – not surprisingly, because their breasts are not getting enough stimulation (see chapter 10). Over the next few weeks they become more and more miserable as they realize their babies are not getting enough to eat and eventually they go out and buy a bottle.

There is no reason why nearly every mother should not breast feed for as long as she wants *provided* she understands how to make enough milk and has enough help.

So in summary, although there are advantages to the breast

feeding mother, none of them is powerful enough to influence a mother who is only concerned with her own well-being. It seems likely that most mothers will decide to breast feed because of the many real advantages to their babies.

6 Preparation and pregnancy

Looking after yourself

We're going to talk here about the things you can do during pregnancy to prepare for breast feeding your baby.

Looking after yourself is important not only for your own sake but for your family's as well. You'll be spending a large part of a year carrying, nourishing and protecting your baby and this is a long time by any standards. It's a good idea now to take care to eat sensibly to maintain your health, prepare your body for breast feeding and provide enough food for your developing baby. It is also sensible to get as much informed ante-natal advice as you can, talk to your husband about your decision to breast feed, get in touch with people who may help you with breast feeding should you run into any problems and generally prepare yourself and your household so that you have as few external problems as possible when you have your new baby.

Choosing your hospital

One of the first things you'll have to do once you know you are pregnant is book into a hospital for your delivery (unless you are going to have a home confinement). Take care when choosing where to have your baby – that is if there is a choice of hospitals in your area – because some hospitals are very much more helpful than others when it comes to breast feeding. In the UK today we are fortunate in having a surplus of maternity beds as a result of the generous provision of beds during the baby boom of the sixties that has now come to an end. This means that many maternity units are short of patients. This is good because it gives you a chance to choose.

If your doctor is not sure which hospital is best, ask other mothers if they were helped with feeding in hospital and what sort of advice they had. If only a few mothers you talk to were completely breast feeding on discharge from your nearest hospital, then go on inquiring until you hear of a hospital where they really do help. Even if this hospital is rather a long way from where you live, it's still almost certainly worth the effort of booking in there if you really want to breast feed. Even the keenest person can be completely discouraged if the hospital allows only rigid schedule feeding, because that gets the establishment of successful breast feeding off to such a bad start.

Another thing to look for is whether the hospital allows or, even better, encourages rooming-in: the practice of having the baby with the mother all the time. This system makes breast feeding much easier and more likely to succeed.

At your booking visit you'll be asked how long you want to stay in after you have had your baby. Times vary throughout the country and some hospitals like you to stay in for longer with a first baby. If you can arrange adequate help at home, you'll almost certainly get more rest at home and you'll also be able to have your baby with you all the time so that you can feed completely on demand, day and night. Mothers who opt for a 48-hour discharge are more likely to breast feed successfully, provided they are given enough help. This is scarcely surprising as these mothers are soon back in their own environment where they can relax. Hospital, after all, is a strange place for most of us and does little to encourage the establishment of the let-down. One American woman logged the number of intruders she had into her private room each day – it came to between fifty and seventy. Some chance of relaxed mothering!

Involving your husband

At some time during your pregnancy you should discuss with your husband what breast feeding is going to mean to him. Make sure that he is as keen for you to breast feed as you are yourself. You can do this by telling him what you have learnt about the advantages of breast feeding, perhaps even giving him this book to read, and taking him to the fathers' night at your ante-natal class, where fathers' doubts and queries can be discussed.

Your husband should be only too pleased to fit in with the baby once he understands how important it is for the baby's feeds to come before him and his mealtimes. Discuss how he is going to get home from the station if you usually pick him up; talk about having supper at a flexible time instead of always on the dot at 7 p.m. and tell him how it'll mean more sleep for you both if you have the baby sleeping with you or next to your bed so that you can feed easily during the night.

Sources of information

Try to find out as much as possible about breast feeding before you actually do it. Even if you have breast fed before – successfully – read about it. You'll find that later there'll be no time for reading and you may be unhappy about the things other people tell you. If you understand how breast feeding works yourself, you'll be much more confident. Remember that all babies are different and the way they feed is totally different too. If you're thoroughly prepared for anything then you'll be more likely to manage.

Your area health authority's ante-natal classes will be valuable and with any luck there'll be a session devoted to baby feeding, a large part of which should be about breast feeding. Try to talk to other mothers there who want to breast feed. Often a film on breast feeding is shown at one of the classes but beware because several of the films in current use give poor advice.

Another source of ante-natal instruction is provided by the National Childbirth Trust which organizes classes throughout the country. A talk from one of their breast feeding counsellors is included at some stage in the course and she will give you her telephone number so that you can contact her if you run into difficulties when breast feeding. Breast feeding counsellors are usually ordinary mothers who have had a short training in counselling for breast feeding problems. They have the advantage over many professionals in that they have almost without exception fed babies themselves and have personal experience of some of the difficulties involved. Your counsellor will be available to talk to you over the phone at any time and will discuss things on a mother-to-mother basis.

You may meet your local health visitor at your ante-natal class. She's the person who is supposed to give you day-to-day support with breast feeding and may well be invaluable when you have your baby back home. Try to find out from other mothers whether she does in fact give good, practical help. If she has the reputation of advising complementary feeds at the drop of a hat, then steer clear of her when your baby is born and go if possible to another baby clinic.

La Leche League International is a world-wide organization of mothers who are breast feeding or who have breast fed their babies and want to help each other and anyone else with problems that may arise with breast feeding. Anyone interested in breast feeding is welcome to attend their meetings.

From about the fifth month, or even before, your breasts will be getting larger and you'll need new bras as your breasts change over the months. A maternity and nursing bra correctly fitted in the last couple of months of pregnancy should give you the right support for the rest of your pregnancy and while breast feeding.

Some women manage to carry on using ordinary bras when breast feeding, undoing them or pulling them down in order to feed – in fact only 40 per cent of breast feeding women buy a special nursing bra. Using ordinary bras can create problems though as it can be difficult to do up a back-fastening bra in a hurry if the doorbell goes when you're feeding. Pulling the bra up or down is not good for your breasts or the bra.

Ideally, it's best either not to wear a bra at all when breast feeding (see page 97), if you have fairly small breasts that don't need the support, or to wear a nursing bra which opens at the front. There are two main types of nursing bra; one has a flap in each cup which opens to reveal the nipple and areola; the other has cups which undo completely at the centre, independently of each other. Beware of the sort of bra that undoes completely in the middle as when undone the two halves spring apart and are difficult to do up again. The centre-opening bra gives good support but takes time to hook up (unless fastened with zips or Velcro). The flap cup bra is very easy to use but unless well fitted it can obstruct milk ducts by pressure from the outer circle of material left when the flap is undone.

You will need several bras as they'll need frequent washing, especially after the birth when you're bound to leak. Some people find cotton more pleasant than nylon because it 'breathes' more. It's important to have the bra fitted well as it should not squash the breasts or nipples at all and it should also provide good support for your breasts. You'll probably want to wear a bra at night because without one you may leak milk over the sheets. Also, because your breasts are heavier they'll probably feel more comfortable when supported at night.

You will need to tuck pads of material or paper nursing pads into your bra to soak up any leaking milk. You can buy paper nursing pads at most chemists. A new pad available soon is shaped like a cone and so stays in place better than the older ones which were flat. Don't use paper tissues or cotton wool because these dry on to the nipples and can be painful to remove. Some women use a square of soft material such as part of an old nappy or cut up pieces of a nappy roll. Avoid plastic-backed pads as they can prevent air from getting to the nipples and so make the skin wet and soggy. The National Childbirth Trust sells a cotton maternity and nursing bra which is available in many different sizes. It is front-opening and does up with laces at the back to allow for change in size during pregnancy and lactation. If you want a pretty nursing bra, many firms make them and they're well worth considering. Neither you nor your husband is going to feel very sexy with you in the average 'sensible' bra that many people suggest.

To get back to your pregnancy, it's probably sensible to wear a good everyday bra in bed for the last three months or so. This will give your breasts the support they need to help ensure they don't get too stretched by their increased weight. After all, if you're worried about losing your figure after having children, now is the time to start caring. The maternity bras sold as sleep bras are usually too insubstantial to provide much support. It's also a good idea to wear a good, firm bra for about six months after the baby has been weaned. This will keep your breasts in good shape as they get back to normal.

Good clothes to buy for breast feeding include blouses, jumpers, T-shirts, anything that will pull up from the waist or do up in front. When it actually comes to feeding a good tip is to undo your bottom buttons to feed and not the top ones. Some women alter their existing clothes to make them more suitable. Make sure you have several changes of clothes because nothing is more depressing than being in the same things day after day. There are lots of nighties available which undo in front and many of these are extremely pretty.

Anything new you buy should be easily washable because apart from your milk leaks, your baby may well regurgitate small amounts of milk over you and dry cleaning bills can mount up very quickly with a new baby in the house.

Furniture

You will probably want to have the baby near you all day so you can hear as soon as he cries. In this case you'll need either a lightweight crib, a cot on wheels or a carrycot to use downstairs. Similarly, if you want to have the baby by your bed at night for easy feeding, it's a good idea to have a readily movable cot to pull over to the bed.

Many baby books talk about buying a special nursing chair and you may think it sounds like a waste of money. A comfortable place to feed the baby is a very real help, though, as it's all too easy to end up after a feed with aching shoulders and arms if you have not been as relaxed as you should be. The chair needs to be low so that your lap is flat to support the baby and it is more comfortable if your elbows are supported by cushions at the right height. Try experimenting with your existing furniture before you have the baby. A rocking chair is often pleasant for both mother and baby. Many mothers find it most comfortable to feed their babies while sitting on a settee or bed with their feet up. Lying down to feed is the most relaxing of all!

Organizing your home

Store as much in the way of food as you can before you have your baby. Stock up with tinned and dried food and if you have a freezer fill it if you can with prepared meals so that you or your husband can rustle up something quickly if necessary when you feel too tired to cook.

If you can afford it, buy stores of things like detergent, nappy sterilizing solution and ordinary household goods. When you're breast feeding, shopping can be a problem at first as the baby may want feeding so often that there isn't much time to go out to do a large shop. You might like to find out whether any local shops deliver, though this seems to be a dying service these days. If you're lucky, your husband may volunteer to go late-night shopping sometimes, or a relative or neighbour may shop for you. This will only be for a few weeks while the baby is really small and feeding very often.

One of the great revelations to a first-time mother is the amount of laundry one small baby can generate. It's worth preparing for this well in advance. If you don't have a washing machine already see if you can possibly afford one now – it'll make all the difference to coping with nappies especially. If you haven't got a machine think about using a laundry for sheets and other big things for the first few weeks you're at home. This is especially important if you come home at forty-eight hours because you may well soil bed clothing with blood or discharge in the first few days.

If the chore of washing nappies without a machine is going to tire you in the early days, treat yourself to a few boxes of disposable nappies. You may find they're too expensive to use after the first week or two but it'll give you a nice easy start while your milk is getting established.

Organizing help at home

When you have your new baby back home, you'll need to take things slowly and easily for a few weeks and this will be much easier if you have someone to help you in the house. This becomes more necessary with a second or third baby, because there's more work with a family of this size. If you haven't any willing relatives nearby, you might like to arrange for a home help to come in daily, though this is rather a luxury. Many husbands take a week or two off work to help out, especially if there are other children. Whatever happens, if you're going to breast feed successfully, you'll need time to do it, especially at first when the baby will need feeding often, so don't put yourself in the role of superwoman.

Nipple and breast care

The advice given routinely to expectant mothers about how to care for their breasts and nipples has done a lot to put many of them off the whole business. The average modern girl and young mum doesn't want to push and poke her breasts and nipples about for months on end before the baby's even born! Mothers have even been heard to say that preparing their breasts for feeding is more fiddly than preparing bottles – so they choose bottles.

There is *no* convincing evidence from all the surveys done so far that any ante-natal care (such as wearing breast shells (shields), rolling the nipples, doing nipple exercises, rubbing the nipples with a rough towel, putting on lanolin, cream or alcohol, expressing colostrum, etc.) *does any good at all*! Having said this, though, we have to admit that there are some women who may be so squeamish that were it not for this breast preparation they might not feed their babies because of their reluctance to handle their own breasts. In these cases breast care might 'decondition' them sufficiently for them to manage breast feeding.

There are three things that *are* worth talking about:

1 *Nipple shape.* Some women have nipples that don't stick out normally but seem to be flat or even inverted. If the areola of a nipple like this is pressed between the finger and thumb, and the nipple then sticks out properly, it's unlikely that the baby will later have any difficulty in sucking. However, if the nipple remains flat or inverted, then there may be some problem with feeding. To get things into perspective, though, 'poor' nipple shape only hinders one in twenty mothers trying to feed their first babies; one in fifty feeding second babies and no mothers who have fed two babies or more.

When the finger-thumb areola test is done ante-natally, it suggests that one in three women pregnant for the first time have 'poor' nipples (either truly inverted or just poorly protractile). So why the discrepancy with the numbers given above? It's because nipple shape and protractility improve spontaneously during pregnancy and this is thought to be because of the action of oestrogens on the tissues behind the nipple.

It's possible you'll be told you should wear breast shells (shields) if your nipples are too flat. These are hollow, plastic or glass, and saucer-shaped with a circular hole on the inner surface for the nipple, and of course they come in pairs. The idea behind them is that by wearing them inside your bra, the nipples will be pressed through the holes and this will improve their shape. They don't show when in position and are usually quite comfortable.

It's doubtful, though, whether wearing breast shells will improve the protractility of the nipples. The nipples that do improve with shells probably would have done so naturally during pregnancy anyway, as we've just described. However, if you have poorly protractile nipples and you're determined to do everything possible to make sure you can feed easily, then wearing breast shells ante-natally inside your bra certainly won't hurt. Breast shells are available on prescription and can be bought over the counter. When ordering or buying, ask for a pair of *breast shields*. We have called them breast shells in the book to differentiate them more clearly from nipple shields, and indeed they are widely known as shells, but they are manufactured under the name of breast shields.

Perhaps a better use for breast shells is after the baby is born, when their use for a time before a feed will often make the nipple protrude enough for the baby to be able to take hold of the breast properly. Obviously, after a few seconds or so the shape of the nipple returns to its original shape, so the baby has to catch hold fairly quickly. The disadvantage of this method is that the shell can obstruct milk ducts because of the pressure it exerts and so can increase the likelihood of engorgement. Also, the nipple skin can become moist and swollen in the shell and so more liable to become sore or cracked.

Many ante-natal clinics routinely look at nipples and advise mothers if they are poorly shaped. However, if they are it's no good just looking, so if someone does this you can be sure that their advice won't be worth listening to. If after doing the finger-thumb test they advise you to wear breast shells, then do so if you want to but remember the benefit from doing so is unproven. If they say your nipples are fine, then at least you'll be reassured. If they don't examine your nipples at all, it shouldn't worry you. If you think your nipples are poorly shaped you can always ask next time and get them to order you breast shells if this would put your mind at rest. Remember that only 5 per cent of first-time mothers have any trouble with their nipples being 'unsuitable' for feeding which is scarcely surprising since this is what they were designed for.

2 *Nipple cleanliness.* The thing to understand here is that the Montgomery's tubercles around the areola secrete a greasy fluid which keeps the skin of the areola and nipple supple and also kills surface bacteria on the skin. If you wash this fluid off with soap, then the skin is much more likely to become sore when you suckle your baby. It doesn't matter how you wash your breasts for most of your pregnancy but keep away from soap for the last few weeks. Just wash your nipples by splashing them with warm water.

There's no need to use any sort of ointment or cream on your nipples to prepare them for breast feeding – Nature's own lubrication is best. Similarly, there's no need to remove any dried secretions from the nipple. A simple water splash is enough.

3 *Expression of milk.* There's no need to express milk ante-natally to remove colostrum or 'clear the ducts' as was once advised. However, it's worth learning the technique even though you won't actually use it now, because it may be useful to know when you've got the baby. (See chapter 7 for details.)

What about all the other things that people tell you to do? It has been shown that 'rolling' the nipples doesn't increase success with feeding. The only reason for doing it would be to make your nipples less sensitive and that will happen anyway once the baby starts feeding. Some women go without their bra or cut a small hole in their bra each side to allow their nipples to rub against their clothing and so become less sensitive. Others rub their nipples with a rough towel each night after their bath, which seems rather hard on them! It also can't be shown to do any good.

So all you need to do is clean your nipples with water alone; learn how to express milk to save you learning later; and if you want to, use breast shells if your nipples are poorly protractile.

Eating the right food

The weight you'll gain during pregnancy is composed of the baby, the placenta, the amniotic fluid and the increased weight of the uterus and breasts, together with the increased amount of blood and other body fluids and stores of fat. Controversy rages over the amount of weight gain considered desirable.

A normal woman eating an unrestricted diet will gain on average twenty-eight pounds during her pregnancy, of which about nine pounds will be made up of fat stores. If she bottle feeds her baby, she may have trouble losing all this excess fat but if she breast feeds, the fat contributes nourishment to the baby via the milk and is used up over the breast feeding period providing she doesn't overeat. Recent research suggests that the fat stores accumulated during pregnancy supply about 300 calories a day to the baby in milk for about three or four months. Given that a baby needs to get around 600–800 calories a day from milk, this means that the breast feeding mother has to eat only 300–500 extra calories a day (provided she has laid down adequate fat stores) in order to provide food for her baby without robbing her own body. This means that the fat she has stored during pregnancy provides between a third and a half of the baby's energy needs. Millions of women in underdeveloped countries don't lay down any fat stores yet still manage to breast feed successfully for long periods.

Many obstetricians advise a weight gain of less than the average twenty-eight pounds and while this may be fine for the bottle feeding mother, the breast feeding mother will have to compensate for her lack of fat stores by eating more while she's breast feeding. Too high a weight gain during pregnancy makes a woman's life more unpleasant though, because she's more likely to have trouble with ankle swelling, varicose veins, backache and heartburn, so don't think that the more weight you put on, the better!

Studies to try and correlate success in breast feeding with the weight gained during pregnancy have yielded conflicting results, one showing that the smaller the amount of fat stored, the greater the amount of milk produced, and another showing that women putting on very little weight during pregnancy had difficulty in feeding their babies. Clearly, more work needs to be done in this field.

So what should you eat? Eat a normal, balanced, healthy diet such as you should eat even when you're not pregnant. There's absolutely no need to eat for two! At the beginning of your pregnancy you may find you want to eat less than usual because of sickness but later you'll probably find that your appetite increases. Overall, you'll need slightly more food than usual to supply the needs of the growing baby and experts suggest a figure of an extra 200 calories a day. However, if like many women you're less active during the last few months of pregnancy, you may not need to eat any more at all.

A normal diet should contain enough protein, fluid, fat, fruit and vegetables and a certain amount of unrefined carbohydrate. Unrefined carbohydrates include wholemeal bread, wholewheat cereals, brown rice and wholemeal flour. Fruit and vegetables should be unpeeled if possible and cooked as little as necessary. Sugar in any form should be avoided as not only is it quite unnecessary for a healthy diet but it is also very high in calories and bad for your teeth. By eating unrefined food you will almost certainly avoid any trouble with constipation – a common problem in pregnancy.

Provided you eat a well-balanced diet, there's no need for you to take any vitamin supplements.

Many people firmly believe that milk is essential for the pregnant woman but this is quite untrue, providing she has enough calcium from other foods and that her diet is adequate overall. Calcium-containing foods include bread, cabbage, watercress, fish and cheese. It's important to take at least some of these foods as the baby needs quite a lot of calcium for bone development and may otherwise rob your own bones of this vital substance. It's important to get this in perspective, though, by looking at many parts of the world where women do not increase their calcium intake during pregnancy and yet have healthy babies and remain healthy themselves. The total body store of calcium in the average healthy woman is more than enough to give the baby all it needs.

It's worth knowing that an expectant mother with two or more children under school age is entitled to seven pints of milk a week free regardless of her family income. Free milk is also available to any expectant mother whose family income is below a certain level.

Many doctors routinely give iron and folic acid supplements to pregnant women. This is to try to prevent the anaemia from deficiency of either of these substances which occurs in a small percentage of pregnant women. The World Health Organization has recommended that there is no need for women in developed countries to take these supplements provided they are eating a balanced diet. Indeed, many women don't take them anyway as the side-effects of iron can be so unpleasant. Routine blood tests should be done during pregnancy (usually at the booking visit and again at thirty-two weeks) to make sure that should true anaemia develop, it can be treated before the baby is born. Old estimates of the numbers of women developing anaemia didn't take into account the fact that the normal woman's haemoglobin concentration in her blood falls during pregnancy as a result of the increased amount of fluid in the blood – this of course is not the same as iron deficiency anaemia. To guard against anaemia you should eat enough foods containing iron (meat, eggs, green vegetables and wholemeal bread) and folic acid (green vegetables, liver, kidneys and yeast).

We'll talk about the ideal diet for a breast feeding mother in chapter 9 but it differs very little from the one we've just described.

So by now you should have everything prepared for breast feeding and be looking forward to the birth of your baby. The next chapter will tell you exactly how to manage from the very first few minutes after birth.

7 The early days

The first few minutes

The moment of birth comes not only at the end of many hours of hard labour but also at the end of nine months' waiting and preparation for the baby's arrival. Not surprisingly, the majority of mothers experience a tremendous sense of physical relief and emotional excitement when the baby is finally born. Feelings of pride at having actually produced a baby that a few hours ago was nothing more than a wriggling bump mingle with fatigue, curiosity and a sense of elation. A few mothers are so exhausted by their labour that all they can think of is having a well-earned rest and unfortunately some are so knocked out by the effects of pain-killing drugs that they can't think of anything at all.

Excessive doses of pain-killers during labour (especially drugs like pethidine) are probably responsible for more breast feeding failure than people have realized. It has been shown that animals anaesthetized while they give birth often reject their young and many mothers say they feel that the baby isn't quite real after giving birth under anaesthetic or under the influence of large amounts of pain-killing drugs. A mother's attachment to her baby will undoubtedly be delayed if she is over-dosed with pain-killing drugs and she will be less likely to breast feed successfully.

Research has shown that those babies born to 'over-doped' mothers don't develop normal feeding patterns until the fourth or fifth day! It's hardly surprising that with a 'difficult feeder' on her hands the mother may become dispirited and give up. See page 152 for some ideas on how to cope.

Here then is a perfect opportunity for your husband to help. He can ensure that you don't get given too much in the way of pain-killers. Only accept another injection if you really need it.

Gas and air is probably a safer way of getting pain relief (from the baby's point of view) than repeated injections of pethidine or similar powerful drugs.

Ideally, a new baby should be handed to his mother straight away to hold and suckle for as long as she wants. If the baby is naked, so much the better, as long as the room is warm enough. Staff permitting, weighing and washing can be done later.

In many obstetric units the newborn baby is wrapped up and handed to the mother to hold for a short time before being weighed, washed and labelled. At the same time, the placenta is delivered and preparations for any stitches are made. It takes a single-minded mother to put her baby to the breast amid all this activity but we strongly recommend that she does because it'll give both her and her baby the best possible start to breast feeding. Some mothers are so delighted with their new babies that immediate suckling seems perfectly normal and not at all embarrassing, even though there is a lot of activity around and it may be the first time they have suckled a baby. Other mothers are not really sure what's expected of them and feel awkward if the baby seems uninterested in the breast.

It has been suggested that the oxytocin secreted by the pituitary into the bloodstream during this first episode of suckling helps expel the placenta and reduce blood loss by its action on the uterus (it makes the muscle fibres contract). Indeed, some primitive peoples use suckling as their only means of encouraging delivery of the afterbirth. If the let-down reflex works – and it will only do so if suckling is continued long enough – then the placenta may be pushed out more quickly but whether or not blood loss is controlled to any extent is doubtful. Anyway, this early suckling is certainly well worth doing, especially because the sucking reflex of a newborn baby is strongest in the first half hour after birth, after which the baby often becomes tired and uninterested in the breast.

Suckling before the umbilical cord is cut has the effect of pushing more blood along the cord into the baby as the uterus contracts. This 'extra helping' of iron-containing blood builds up the iron stores of the baby and so has much to recommend it.

It has been shown in four separate worldwide studies that early contact with her newborn baby makes a mother more likely to breast feed successfully and also increases the length of time she'll continue to feed. It seems that there is a 'sensitive period' probably lasting about twelve hours which is crucial to the development of mother-child bonding. If the mother and child are separated for this period then the mother's behaviour towards the child may differ not only with respect to breast feeding but also in the amount of affection she shows on the second day. All this means that the priority shouldn't be to take the baby away and give the mother time to sleep but should be to let mother and baby be together. A mother's sleep is more likely to be deep if she has looked at, cuddled and suckled her baby than if she is worrying about where he is and what is happening to him.

Have a good look at your baby and enjoy your first meeting. You may well not feel any rush of motherly love – many mothers say that this takes time to come – but at least you'll be curious to examine and touch him. Uncover your breast one side and see if your baby wants to feed. If he does, then let him carry on as long as he wants. If he doesn't want to, *don't worry*. He will soon enough. It's all too easy to be discouraged by a baby that doesn't seem very interested but remember that he doesn't yet know why he should suck. When he has tasted your colostrum he'll be much keener!

What's the best way to put the baby to the breast? If you're lying down, roll to one side and lay the baby down by you so that he's on his side with his head facing your breast. Then stroke his cheek or the corner of his mouth with your nipple. He'll probably open his mouth as he turns towards the nipple and then start feeding when he finds it. This searching movement is called *rooting* and is an inborn reflex in newborn babies. Don't hold his head or push it towards the breast or he'll turn his mouth towards the pressure of your hand and that will be the opposite way from the way you want him to turn!

If you can sit up comfortably, then hold the baby in the crook of one arm, make sure you're comfortable, preferably with your elbow supported, and do what we've just described. If the baby is comfortable, with his whole body facing yours, not just with his head turned to your breast, then he's more likely to feed.

Don't worry if you feel inexperienced or at a loss how to hold and behave with your baby. This is quite normal, especially if it's your first time. Nurses and doctors may imply that you should know instantly how to be a perfect mother. This is unfair and can be especially hurtful at this time. Studies with animals show that they too need time and experience to become good at mothering. Some zoo animals need to be taught how to 'mother' by male keepers!

So far we've been talking about the average mother who has had a normal labour. This doesn't always happen, though, and we'll talk about the mother who has had a Caesarian section or other problems in chapter 13.

So what happens next? Ideally, if you, your husband and your baby are all content, the staff should leave you together for a while – perhaps half an hour or so. After that you'll be washed and given clean things to wear and the baby can have all the necessary routine things done. You and the baby will most likely feel tired out – labour is tough not only for you but for your baby too – and you'll both want a good sleep.

Rooming-in

Enlightened hospitals allow the baby to sleep in your bed or in a cot by you and be with you all the time, knowing that you'll sleep better and be happier with your baby by you day and night. Studies show that mothers who have their babies with them are twice as likely to succeed at breast feeding than if their babies are in a nursery. After all, you've had him with you for nine months and there's no good reason to take him away now. The only exception may be if you're in a large ward where having all the babies in by their mothers at night might keep everyone awake. In this case it may be better to let the babies stay in the nursery and for the nurses to bring them in to their mothers for feeding when they cry. Although it is still a rare occurrence, some hospitals allow mothers to have their babies in bed with them all the time. This works very well for mothers, babies and the nursing staff, even in a large ward.

In general it's fair to say that no hospital can possibly have enough staff to give the kind of love and care that the baby's mother can give. It's scarcely surprising then that babies who room-in are more contented than those kept in nurseries and brought to their mothers occasionally.

If you feel very strongly about having your baby with you at night but the hospital staff are not keen, then ask your husband to discuss it with them. If *you* make a fuss you may get upset.

Breast milk only

If your baby is taken away from you, you must insist that he is brought to you for feeding as soon as he cries and that he must *not be given anything to drink*, even if it's only water or sugar water. Don't be fobbed off with explanations or excuses – he's your baby and as we've already explained earlier in this chapter, the best way to establish successful lactation is to feed him frequently in the first few days. If he has anything else to drink, he won't want to feed at the breast.

Many mothers have described the agony they went through when they could hear their babies crying and yet weren't allowed to have them brought to them. What nurses often don't understand is that a mother doesn't know the sound of her baby's voice this soon after birth and so worries every time *any* baby cries. She'll have far more peace of mind with her baby by her. Her milk will also come in far sooner if she picks up the baby to feed him not only whenever he cries but also whenever she wants to.

Ill-informed nurses and midwives will ask why it is that *your* baby is not allowed to drink cows' milk, sugar water or boiled water at night (or when you are asleep) when every other baby has it and seems to get on well enough. If you feel that you must explain, then tell her that there are many reasons why breast milk alone is best. If it makes things easier, here's a list.

1 Your breasts need to be emptied frequently to produce plenty of milk. Infrequent feeding will diminish your milk supply.

2 The more your baby feeds, the sooner your milk will come in.

3 Your baby needs colostrum to protect him from infection, to

give him the foods he needs in the correct proportions and to supply him with immunoglobulins and other substances not present in cows' milk.

4 Your baby shouldn't have cows' milk because it contains 'foreign' protein which might sensitize him and so predispose to allergy later.

5 He shouldn't have cows' milk because this would satiate his appetite for several hours and so make him less likely to want breast milk. The bottle fed baby goes longer between feeds than the breast fed baby because cows' milk takes longer to be digested.

6 He shouldn't have sugar water because there's a chance that it may harm his pancreas by stimulating the outflow of insulin too early in life. Your own milk will provide all the sugar and water he could possibly need. A high calorie drink would anyway satiate his appetite and once again prevent him from wanting to feed at the breast. A sudden slug of sugar is completely unphysiological and unnatural, so why give it?

7 Properly breast fed babies don't need water. Your breast milk has enough even in the first days.

8 He shouldn't be fed with a bottle and a teat. A rubber teat is so easy for the baby to drink from and provides such a strong stimulus to suck that the baby may be loath to return to your breast when he finds he has to work harder to get his milk from you.

Hospitals sometimes used to recommend that all babies had water or sugar water as their first drink in case there was a congenital abnormality of their windpipe and gullet and milk was inhaled. This is now no longer justified.

Night feeds

During your hospital stay it's ideal if your baby can be in your bed or in a cot by you at night but if he has to go into a nursery then make sure that you tell the nurses each night that you are breast feeding. Although they should know, it's easy to get a young nurse who is inexperienced, an agency nurse who is new or a nurse who, thinking she is doing you a favour, will not bring your baby to you to be fed but will give him a bottle along with all the other bottle fed babies at 2 a.m. Some mothers who have been warned about this write out a card which they tie on to their baby's cot. The card says 'I am breast fed – please take me to my mother when I cry.' This won't upset anybody and will probably make it easier for you to get your own way. It's worth getting yourself mentally geared up to night feeds because you'll be doing plenty of them. Night feeds may decrease from two months or so but many babies are loath to give them up for several months.

Natural breast feeding

Feed your baby whenever he cries; seems to want feeding; when your breasts are full; and more often if you want to. *Don't feed on any sort of schedule.* The more schedule feeding there has been this century, the fewer breast feeding mothers there have been. Schedules reduce the likelihood of successful breast feeding. We've already shown why this is so in chapter 2. However, while demand feeding works perfectly well for many mothers and their babies, it's not necessarily the best way of feeding a baby because he may not ask for enough feeds. In this case your milk supply will dwindle. Natural breast feeding doesn't mean waiting until your baby asks – you may want to feed him at other times because your breasts are full, because you're going out or because you just want to cuddle him. In any case, don't leave your baby unfed for more than three hours at the longest – longer gaps will endanger your milk supply and may mean your baby is not getting enough food. Some mothers find their babies go as long as four or five hours between some feeds but as a general rule this is not sensible in the early days.

Demand feeding is usually held to be the ideal form of breast feeding – which it certainly is when compared with schedule feeding. But it's still not as good as natural breast feeding where both mother's and baby's needs are met whenever they want.

Babies gain weight better when fed on demand because their mothers produce more milk when they feed frequently. Many people have worked out the average number of feeds demanded by babies each day after birth and this number varies a lot, according to the individual baby. Don't worry about the number of feeds your baby has compared with the demand fed baby in the next bed – it doesn't matter and is no indication of the success you'll have. All babies are different.

So for that matter are mothers. Don't compare yourself with the other women around you even if they're breast feeding. Obviously it's interesting to know how many feeds your neighbour's baby has but the danger is that you'll start competing with each other. This is one reason why mothers breast feed more successfully if they go home soon after delivery.

You'll probably find that the nurses and midwives on your ward will be unwilling to let you feed on demand because it doesn't fit into their routine. Persist as much as you feel is reasonable. If it'll help you, tell them that research in a hospital in Oxford found that the nurses' work fell dramatically when they changed from schedule to demand breast feeding.

Babies allowed absolutely unrestricted access to their mothers' breasts – for example those carried next to a naked breast all day in some underdeveloped countries – don't have to cry before they are fed. These babies feed *very much more often* than babies fed even completely on demand in the Western world. This is true natural breast feeding.

Some mothers worry about waking their babies during the daytime in order to feed them. You ought to wake him if it's a long time since a feed or if your breasts are feeling full. If you don't you'll regret it (and so will he in the end) because your breasts will become tense or even truly engorged and your milk production will slow down. Your baby will soon go back to sleep again so don't worry. After all, you're a nursing pair – sometimes you'll feed for his benefit and sometimes for yours. As the weeks go by your supply will tune in to his demand but in the meantime a few extra feeds will do no harm. As a general rule, you should *never* go so long between feeds that your breasts feel tense and lumpy.

Finally, mothers of naturally breast fed babies are only half as likely to get sore nipples as those of schedule fed babies.

How long should you feed?

You'll almost certainly be told to feed your baby for a specified number of minutes each side and to increase the time each day until the fifth day when you'll be 'allowed' ten minutes a side. This restriction of feeding time is not only completely unnatural but will hinder your milk from coming in; may not give your let-down reflex time to work and become established; will prevent your baby from getting as much colostrum as he could get and will make you much *more* likely to get sore nipples. This has all been known for years but some hospitals still insist on out-of-date rules.

Babies, like adults, want different amounts of food day by day and even within any given day. Sometimes your baby will want a snack and other times a feast. Research done recently in southern Africa has shown that any given baby feeding on demand will take meals of very different volumes at different times (sometimes a tenfold difference)

If you're not the sort of person to make a fuss, and few women are when they've just had a baby, then go ahead and suckle for as long as you want anyway.

Let your baby feed till he's had enough. Once he loses interest in the first breast, change him to the second. Always try to feed from both breasts in the early days or the unemptied one will produce less milk because of back-pressure on the milk-producing cells.

Start the next feed with the breast you fed with last because the let-down is more efficient early in a breast feed. The first breast is therefore usually emptied better than the second and it's important for both breasts to take turns at being completely emptied.

How to tell when he's had enough

Many babies show they've had enough simply by falling asleep but before that stage a baby may well unclench his fists, smile, show obvious refusal or arch his back. Don't force him to feed more. Learn to accept your baby's judgement of what he wants. After a while you'll get to know how much he's had by feeling your breasts. If they're soft he's probably had all there is.

Crying

There's an awful lot going on in the average maternity ward, what with trolley shops, paper rounds, meals, visitors, bed-making and room cleaning, to say nothing of doctors' and nurses' rounds, flowers to arrange, letters and cards to open and send, baths, talking to your neighbour in the next bed and so on. It's all too easy to let the baby come second while you go on doing whatever you were doing when he started crying. Remember that if you leave him crying for long, he'll get tired out because infants expend a lot of energy in crying – just look and you'll see why. When your baby has been crying for a long time you'll probably find he doesn't feed well – he has literally exhausted himself with crying and hasn't got the strength to feed.

Obviously a minute or so of crying won't hurt, but try not to let it go on much longer.

At first you won't have a clue why he's crying and this can make any new mother feel inadequate but it's the only way he can communicate. After a few weeks you may be able to distinguish his cries between demands for nappies, food, sleep and so on.

Long periods of crying are one of the main reasons why babies fed on a four-hourly schedule don't get enough breast milk and why their mothers often fail with breast feeding. A baby who wakes an hour early and is left to cry until the clock says it is time for a feed won't be hungry when feed time arrives – he'll just be tired out. Over a few days his mother's breasts won't have been stimulated enough because she won't have suckled enough so there won't be enough prolactin and oxytocin released (see chapter 2) and her milk supply will fail.

There are two other reasons why babies shouldn't be left to cry. Firstly, no mother likes to hear her baby crying – crying means unhappiness to most people. This will upset her even if she pretends it doesn't and her let-down reflex (see chapter 2) may easily be suppressed as a result.

Secondly, it seems sensible to comfort a squawling infant straight away as this will encourage him to think that mother is good and that the world is a good place to be in. You can't possibly spoil a baby like this. If you were left to yell for hours for your food you would be angry with the person who was stopping you from eating.

The ability to comfort her crying baby at the breast is one of the greatest pleasures for the breast feeding mother. If she limits suckling time this pleasure will be denied both her and her baby. Breast feeding is not only a means of getting milk, it's also a way of being close to a warm, soft, comforting mother.

How to hold the baby

If you can, experiment with various positions by yourself. If you've got someone who is in a hurry or unsympathetic standing by you, pushing and prodding the baby, neither you nor your baby will be relaxed and the feed is unlikely to go well. We've talked briefly about feeding the baby sitting up or lying down after delivery. The main things are to make yourself comfortable (because you'll be in the same position for some time) and to get the baby comfortable. Try supporting the baby's weight with a pillow on your lap. Another pillow under your supporting arm might help. If you're sitting it's easier if you are sitting upright and perhaps leaning forward slightly. Try holding the baby with his chest and tummy against you so that he doesn't have to turn his head round but can feed with his head straight. Some babies like it best if they have something to hold on to – try giving him your finger. Many mothers find that as soon as their baby has had enough he lets go of whatever he's holding.

Don't push his mouth on to your nipple as the rooting reflex will make him turn away towards your hand. Just stroke the side of his mouth with your nipple and offer him the nipple in your hand and with luck he'll latch on. Some babies have such a strong rooting reflex that they turn their heads to feed even if a sheet or some clothing touches their cheek. Others need help to get them latched on. If your breast is very full you may have to hold it back so that his nose isn't smothered, otherwise don't bother to hold your nipple or breast once he's feeding. Expressing a little milk from a full breast will soften it enough to enable the baby to latch on.

Your nipple and as much of the areola as possible should be

taken into the baby's mouth as the milk reservoirs are under the areola and need to be emptied by the baby's mouth movements. If only the nipple goes in, not enough milk will be drawn out and because the baby is not getting enough he'll suck very strongly and may make your nipples sore. If you have a large areola which the baby finds difficult to take into his mouth, try holding it between your finger and thumb and squeezing them together. This will make the areola flatter and easier for him to take. A good principle is to aim the nipple at the baby's nose once it's in his mouth – this will ensure it's in the best position (high up in the mouth) and will not get hurt when he sucks on it.

But most important of all is to relax as you feed. Think back to your relaxation teaching from ante-natal classes and relax every muscle you can. Enjoy your baby as he feeds – many mothers experience a very real sense of physical pleasure. Don't let anything put you off this happy, relaxed state of mind. If you're happier with curtains drawn round the bed, ask someone to draw them for you. If anyone makes adverse comments about the baby not feeding well, tell them calmly that you've got all the time in the world to learn. Remember that a baby can safely go the first few days without much to drink – Nature only intended him to have small amounts of colostrum from you.

A difference you may notice between your baby and a bottle fed one is that your baby doesn't feed continuously. Your baby may stop feeding every so often and look around. This is because the let-down causes milk to be spurted into the ducts and from the nipple in an uneven flow. Several spurts of milk come out and then there is a short pause before milk is again ejected. Your baby is just adapting to the flow of your milk. His breathing pattern is also altered to fit in with this drinking pattern.

What about stopping him feeding?

Some babies simply let the nipple go when they've had enough to drink whilst others have to be gently removed from the breast or they'll be there all day.

Never pull a baby's mouth away from the breast while he's feeding. This can damage the nipple and areola as the strong negative pressure is broken. It is better to break the pressure by putting the tip of your little finger in the corner of his mouth. He will then come easily and painlessly away from the nipple.

What is he getting?

At first your baby gets colostrum which provides him with many essential nutrients. This colostrum gradually changes into mature milk during the first few days. There is no sudden change. The more a baby feeds the sooner milk will be produced in large amounts and when this happens it's known as the milk 'coming in'. In a mother feeding her baby frequently, the milk may come in on the second or third day after birth. In a mother feeding her baby infrequently, it may not come in until the fourth or fifth day. Obviously the sooner the milk comes in, the sooner the baby will get plenty to drink. The mother having her second baby will find that her milk comes in sooner than it did with her first.

The phrase 'the milk coming in' is misleading in that it has led many people to think that before the milk comes in, the breasts are empty. Of course they aren't, as you can see if you express some colostrum. Colostrum is only produced in fairly small amounts. It's meant to be this way and even very small volumes are worth their weight in gold to the baby. So valuable is colostrum in protecting the newborn baby against infections (among other things) that some experts believe that every bottle fed baby should receive a 'colostrum cocktail'. Farmers have been giving this to their valuable cattle for years.

Engorgement

When the milk comes in you should carry on feeding your baby completely on demand so that you avoid getting engorged breasts. Mothers feeding their babies on schedule are twice as likely to suffer from engorgement as those feeding on demand. If you are feeding your baby the natural way you'll never get engorged.

Mothers who notice a large increase in the size of their breasts when their milk comes in often think that their milk supply must be failing when their breasts become smaller. However, the supply isn't failing (providing they are feeding their babies on demand), it's just that the breasts often revert to a smaller size once the milk supply equals the demand.

Expressing your milk

You may need to express some milk by hand in the first few days in hospital while your baby's needs are catching up with your supply and certainly it's a useful technique to know for later just in case you need it. If you do become at all engorged, then it may be difficult for the baby to grasp the nipple and areola as the breast is so tense. Expressing some milk will soften the breast enough to allow him to latch on.

If your baby is premature and so too immature to breast feed, milk will have to be given via a tube. You can establish your milk by expressing milk at regular intervals – preferably every two to three hours – and this can be given to your baby by tube.

To express milk, hold the areola between your thumb and first finger. Some people find it easier to use the left hand for both breasts and use the right hand to collect the milk in a container. Move your hand firmly backwards towards your chest. Now move your hand away, pressing your finger and thumb together, so gently squeezing milk out of the milk reservoirs under the areola. Even when milk is expressed it's still necessary for your let-down reflex to work for the hindmilk to be obtained. The milk will then come in spurts with intervals between and you should go on expressing even during the intervals to stimulate the let-down. Many women also massage the whole breast gently to encourage milk flow.

Expressing milk often takes longer than actually feeding the baby but is easy once you have the knack. Don't worry if you can only express a small amount. Many successful breast feeders can never express more than one or two ounces.

Having expressed the milk into a sterile bottle, put a cap on the bottle and keep it in the fridge. Many people say you can freeze milk but this must harm the valuable living cells so don't keep it in the freezer unless it is the only way you can store it safely. Frozen breast milk is still much better than cows' milk.

Nipple care
Wash your nipples with water *but not* soap when you have a bath. If you are told to put salt in the water to help heal your perineum, don't worry, just splash your breasts with plain water to remove the salt before you dry them. Don't let your nipples soak in the water as this will make them more liable to soreness and cracking.

There's no need to put anything on your nipples. Although lanolin or special creams such as Massé cream won't hurt, they are unnecessary as Montgomery's tubercles provide natural secretions.

There's no need to wash your breasts and nipples before you feed. By all means wash them after if you want to, to remove traces of milk, but only do so with water and then dry them well.

The nipple skin can easily become soggy and liable to crack if it's left moist. Avoid this by changing your breast pads often, by using a 'one-way' nappy liner instead of a conventional breast pad or best of all by leaving your bra off altogether so that your nipples are open to the air.

This advice may sound rather complicated – all you need to do in fact is wash your breasts with water only and keep the nipples dry between feeds. That's all!

Nipple soreness and pain
Quite a few mothers experience soreness of their nipples during the first week or perhaps later. This seems to affect fair-skinned women with pale areolae more than darker-skinned women with dark areolae. Unfortunately, the pain makes many mothers give up breast feeding – often because they're given wrong advice on how to cope with it.

By looking after your nipples as we've described above and by feeding naturally you may be able to prevent the onset of soreness. If you can't, then turn to chapter 12 for details of what to do.

Sleeping
Try and get as much sleep as you can during the first few days

especially as labour is a tiring experience for most mothers and broken nights also take their toll.

The nursing staff may suggest that you rest lying on your tummy for an hour or so every day. This position is uncomfortable if your breasts are at all full but you can make yourself quite comfy if you lie with your head on one pillow with another pillow below your breasts so as to make a sort of bridge.

Visiting

This can be a vexed subject. You feel left out if you don't have visitors when everyone else does; you want to show off your new baby to your relatives and friends; you may feel shy about feeding in front of people but yet don't want your baby to go hungry if he cries at visiting times; and a whole hour may be too much for you with some visitors but not enough with others.

There are several ways to cope. Try and choose a hospital that allows fairly unrestricted visiting and then get your husband to vet all the people who want to come and see you. If you wouldn't feel happy about feeding in front of them, get him to put them off, tactfully, of course. There'll be plenty of other opportunities to see them.

Doing this will mean that you won't have to worry if your baby wants a feed during visiting – you'll just go ahead and do it. When people come to see you at home you can always go to another room to feed if you're shy, but you can't do that in hospital.

Nappy changing

Many hospitals advise changing the baby's nappy before a feed. This is all very well if the baby isn't screaming his head off but if he is, wait till the end of the feed otherwise you'll be so upset you may not let down your milk. Some babies don't feed well with a wet or dirty nappy and changing after a feed might wake them – this is why changing before a feed is suggested. But after a good feed most babies are so content and full that nothing, not even a nappy change, will wake them. If you have one of those babies who won't feed in a dirty nappy, you'll soon find out and will have to change him first.

A change after a feed would seem to make more sense because babies nearly always wet or mess their nappies during a feed. For the baby who falls asleep halfway through a feed a nappy change will often wake him enough to take the second breast.

Baby's bowels

A breast fed baby's motions gradually change during the first week from the dark green meconium of the first day or so to bright yellow, liquid motions which may only be seen as a stain on the nappy. Contrast this with a bottle fed baby who has bulky motions almost as soon as he has got rid of the meconium.

Wind

Why haven't we mentioned winding yet? Because many breast fed babies don't need winding – they simply bring up any wind quite spontaneously or pass it out the other end. If you think he's windy, cuddle him in a fairly upright position after a feed to let the wind come up. If you know that your baby doesn't usually burp, you can lay him down to sleep immediately after a feed. Wind is a subject that seems to have become an obsession with British mothers. Many countries of the world, including some European ones, don't recognize wind as being a problem and so do nothing about it.

Colic

Many babies cry for long periods during the day and especially in the evenings during the first three months. This crying is traditionally put down to 'evening colic' or 'three month colic' as it is also known. It is generally assumed that the 'colic' is caused by excess gas in the baby's bowels causing pain as it is passed through. There is, however, no evidence to prove that this is so and it is highly likely that these bouts of crying are not due to colic at all. Other explanations include the baby being upset because his mother is overwrought with the evening rush of things to do – babies quickly sense and respond to moods; the baby being hungry because he is schedule fed and only allowed ten minutes each side, even if his mother hasn't as much milk as at other feeds because she is tired; and lastly, the baby may just want attention and cuddling at the very time of day when his mother can't give it.

The best way to cope with 'colic' is to relax and reduce the amount of work you are doing; feed the baby as much as he wants and just sit and cuddle him if he is happier like that. Drug treatment should then be unnecessary.

Regurgitation

Many babies, especially small ones, regurgitate milk during and after a feed, especially if the milk flow from the breast is very fast or if they are overfilled. Sometimes a baby will bring up so much curdled milk that he will want more to drink to replace it! There is no need to worry if your baby is thriving yet regurgitates milk like this. If your milk flow is very fast at first, though, you might try expressing some milk before feeding your baby, to prevent him drinking it too quickly.

Afterpains

When your let-down reflex works, you may notice low tummy pains which are caused by oxytocin making your womb contract. It means not only that your womb is being encouraged to return to its former size but also that your let-down is working, which is heartening to know. Other signs that your let-down is working are tingling in the breasts, dripping or spraying of milk, the relief of nipple pain when the milk gets to the baby and the swallowing noises the baby makes.

Talking of pains, don't hesitate to tell the doctors or nurses if you're getting pain from episiotomy stitches, piles or whatever. There's nothing like a nagging pain from any source to put the dampers on the let-down reflex. Today you don't have to grin and bear it. Try something simple first like a hot bath and then ask for a rubber ring to sit on to take the weight off the most tender parts. If these don't work, ask for some pain-killers.

Leaking

This obviously happens if your let-down works before the baby is put to the breast but happens even without the let-down if your breasts are full, and especially if you are warm. Leaking means that your breasts are full and ready for the baby and ideally you should suckle your baby so as to relieve them, even if he doesn't seem hungry. If your breasts are full too long, they're highly likely to become engorged in the first few weeks.

If you do leak don't worry that you're producing too much milk – you're not. Don't cut down on your fluid intake in an effort to stop leaking as this will not help. You can cope with leaking by using breast pads, soft material such as a hanky, an old nappy cut into squares or a folded 'one-way' nappy liner tucked into your bra. A trick many mothers have discovered is to put the heel of one hand over the nipple and push in firmly towards the breast. This often stops the leaking like magic. To avoid soaking your nipple in soggy material while feeding from the first breast, try uncovering the second breast and letting the leaking milk drip on to a nappy. Soggy nipple skin, especially in the first few weeks, can make soreness and cracking much more likely.

Baby blues

Many newly delivered mothers feel weepy and emotional towards the end of the first week. This often coincides with the milk coming in and may be the result of the surging changes in hormones. It happens just as often in bottle feeding mothers. Unfortunately, if a mother is having any trouble feeding her baby, this temporary depression may be the last straw that makes her decide to change to the bottle.

Apart from hormonal changes, it's not surprising that a newly delivered mother is emotional. Giving birth is a crisis point in a woman's life and the accompanying loss of sleep and the excitement surrounding a new baby are bound to upset even the calmest person to some extent. It's not uncommon for one mother in a ward to start crying and for all the others to follow suit. All the more reason then to learn how to breast feed before you have your baby, so at least you haven't got that to worry about.

To add to all these perfectly normal things, modern hospital procedures that institutionalize and regiment the new mother do nothing to help. The baby blues are undoubtedly made all the worse for those mothers whose babies are taken away from them and kept in nurseries. Having your baby with you will make you a whole lot happier.

Normal weight loss

A newborn baby has a lot of fluid in his body to tide him over the first few days when his mother's colostrum doesn't provide much volume.

The weight loss that is a perfectly normal occurrence in the first few days occurs because of the loss of this fluid. Most babies lose 6 per cent of their body weight and many lose 10 per cent.

Weight gain

The speed at which a breast fed baby regains his birth weight depends to some extent on whether he is fed on demand or not. Babies fed on demand don't lose much weight after birth and have a more rapid weight gain than babies on a three-hourly feeding schedule. Babies on a three-hourly schedule do better than those on a four-hourly one.

In one study, 49 per cent of demand fed babies and 36 per cent of four-hourly fed babies had regained their birth weight by a week. The demand fed babies in this particular survey were, however, restricted in their number of feeds for the first two days; had they not been, there might have been even more babies regaining their birth weight at one week in this group.

But the speed at which birth weight is regained is not very important. In the old days a mother was not allowed to take her baby home until it had regained its birth weight! Amazingly enough, this still sometimes happens today. Provided that the baby is feeding at least on demand; seems happy; that his weight is slowly rising and the mother's let-down reflex is working and that the nappy is wet when it is changed at each feed, then the rate of weight gain is unimportant. Many breast fed babies take three weeks or more to regain their birth weight. Do *not* give complementary feeds. This will reduce the amount of breast milk available because the baby won't want to eat so much and the feeding stimulus is essential for milk production. *Complementary feeds should not be allowed* by the mother who wants to breast feed successfully. As one mother said, 'How can supply and demand work if you suppress half the demand?'

If there is any doubt as to whether your baby is thriving, increase your milk supply by feeding him more often. (See chapter 10 for details.)

Enlightened hospitals have stopped test weighing babies routinely. Test weighing in most cases only worries people unnecessarily; it worries the staff who think a breast fed baby needs the same volume of milk as a bottle fed baby and it worries the mother because she automatically doubts her ability to feed her baby. Test weighing should be reserved for those babies who are obviously not thriving.

We haven't talked so far about the mother who has her baby at home, mainly because if she has enough help everything will be very much easier for her. Hospitals are safe places to have babies but they are not ideal when it comes to breast feeding. Similarly, we haven't mentioned the mother who is discharged home early. Breast feeding is more successful in both these groups of mothers – a fact that hospital midwives would do well to remember. To try to remedy this state of affairs, some hospitals now have lactation nurses whose sole job is to encourage breast feeding mothers. With enough help from these specialists, longer stays in hospital need not necessarily mitigate against successful feeding.

Feeding your baby in these first days in hospital is a somewhat unnatural and often difficult experience. After all, so much of ward routine does nothing to help the breast feeding mother. As soon as you and the baby are well enough you should be at home in your own environment.

8 Feeding day by day

Going home

Taking your baby home is an exciting occasion whether or not it's your first. However tempting it is to rush around in hospital making both yourself and the baby look nice for your husband to collect, it's sensible not to overdo it because the last thing you want is to arrive home tired out.

Once you get home, sit down and have a cup of tea and just relax. Leave the washing up, ironing and tidying to someone else for a few days if you possibly can. You'll have your hands quite full enough with the baby. All too often a mother plunges back into her old routine and quickly becomes exhausted. Then when her milk dwindles she's surprised and upset and a vicious circle is set up. For the next few weeks you should relax, eat a nourishing diet and let the world go by as much as possible.

If you have your baby at home or if you are discharged early from hospital, this advice is doubly important. It's unlikely that you would even be allowed to contemplate having a home delivery or an early discharge if your doctor and midwife were not sure you had enough help in the home.

Of course, not every baby is a first baby and you may have other children to look after. Hopefully, you and your husband will have made some arrangements with a relative, friend or paid help to come and help out in the first few weeks. Some husbands arrange time off to be at home but this is rarely enough. Many local authorities in this country can supply home helps who will come and do almost anything domestic you need done. You pay them at a reasonable commercial rate but if you are on a very low income you can apply for financial help. Your mother is often the best person to help but nowadays mothers are not always close at hand. Needless to say if your mother is anti-breast feeding you'll have to handle the situation especially carefully if you're going to succeed.

A helper figure or 'doula' as she is called is a very important member of society in many parts of the world where breast feeding is widely practised. Besides giving practical help she often provides emotional support in the first crucial days. Her very presence in the home makes things easier because new mothers tend to worry over tiny things at first and on-the-spot reassurance from someone sympathetic is a godsend.

Whatever sort of help you think you'll need, discuss it with your helper before the baby is born so that you both know where you stand. A problem can sometimes crop up if the helper wants to look after the baby and expects you to look after the house and other children. Clear this sort of matter up as tactfully and quickly as possible. It's worth deciding whether you are going to feed the baby in front of your helper or not and such things are easier to decide before the time comes, to avoid hurting anyone's feelings.

How long should your helper stay? This is an individual decision for every mother but remember that your milk supply may take many weeks to become properly 'established' and you'll need time to recover from the physical effort of pregnancy and labour. So don't rush her departure, especially if you have more than one child. Make the most of any willing help there may be.

Where to feed

Although in theory you can feed your baby anywhere, you'll find it more pleasurable if you are comfortable. If you find you like cushions to support your arm or the baby, make sure they are left in the chair you use. Having said this, though, there's absolutely no need to make a big thing about certain numbers of cushions, chair height and so on. One woman told us that she stopped breast feeding because she couldn't bear all the fiddling with cushions! Many mothers find it most relaxing and enjoyable to feed their babies when lying down on a bed or a settee.

If your baby is a winter baby, remember that you may feel cold when feeding, so keep the room warm. Cold air can make the muscle fibres in the areolae and nipples contract and so delay the release of milk. This may frustrate the baby early in a feed. In practice, the warmth of the baby's mouth will warm the nipples and the let-down reflex will make the skin of the breasts feel warm.

If you find you like something to do while you're feeding, keep a book by your chair. One mother we know found a music stand invaluable for holding her book, so leaving her hands free. You may find it relaxing to watch the television or listen to the radio, though many mothers are quite happy just to watch their baby feeding, especially if he stares up at them as so many babies do. A lot will depend on how long the feed takes – if your baby is a quick feeder, you won't get bored. Feeding should be a time you look forward to and enjoy; if you take care of your own creature comforts, you'll relax, the baby will get the milk easily and everything should go well. In fact, many nursing mothers look forward to feed times as oases of peace in their day.

If on the other hand you perch on a hard chair to feed, with shoulders aching from supporting the baby's weight and dreading the thought of up to an hour's stint with nothing to do other than look at the baby, it's unlikely that you'll relax, the milk won't let down and your baby will go hungry.

Many mothers find they get very thirsty when feeding, especially in the first few weeks. If you do, get yourself something to drink before you start so as to avoid interrupting the feed.

Where to keep your baby during the day

If you put your baby in his room to sleep during the day, you run the risk of not hearing when he wakes. Try keeping him sleeping in a carry cot in the room where you are. That way you'll know when he wakes and will be able to nurse him as soon as he cries. Household noise is unlikely to keep him awake if he really wants to sleep, and if he doesn't it'll be more interesting for him to watch and listen to what's going on than to lie in a quiet room gazing at the ceiling. Having said this, there's no reason to put your baby in a cot between feeds. Many babies are most content when they are carried around in a baby sling for most of the day.

How often?

We feel that more misleading advice has been given about this than about anything else to do with breast feeding and that this advice has done a lot of harm to breast feeding over the past fifty years or more.

Your baby is unlike any other baby – he's an individual and not just a stomach to be filled every three or four hours by the clock. His only way of telling you he is hungry is by crying, given that in this country we don't carry our babies by our naked breasts so that they can feed when they want without even asking. Some mothers swear they can separate their babies' cries into hunger cries, wet and dirty cries, bored cries and so on. We think that this is unlikely in the first few weeks, when all cries sound pretty much the same to the new mother. The only way to decide whether his cry is a 'hungry' one is to offer him the breast. As young babies prefer to have frequent small feeds, he'll almost certainly drink. This is what is known as feeding on demand – *any cry should be interpreted as a request for food until proven otherwise.* There may be the odd occasion when he is clearly not interested in feeding but almost every time he will be. When he's content, then change his nappy if necessary.

Don't be misled by all the advice you are bound to be given from friends, relatives, professionals, baby feeding pamphlets from cows' milk manufacturers and old-fashioned baby books. Many of these sources of information include the old chestnuts about feeding the baby every four hours (2 a.m., 6 a.m., 10 a.m., 2 p.m., 6 p.m. and 10 p.m.). This advice 'is for the birds' and bottle fed babies, not for you and your baby! Some women can probably cope with such a routine but many find their milk supply slowly dwindles simply because six feeds a day don't give the breasts enough stimulation in these vital early weeks.

Once you accept that your baby may ask for feeds very erratically, you're halfway towards feeding successfully. If you worry each time he asks for a feed within an hour of being fed, you're on the path to losing your milk, as worry tends to prevent the let-down reflex from working.

During these early weeks you may find you seem to be spending a large part of the day feeding your baby. That may well be but it's worth accepting and enjoying it and not resenting it.

Although many babies establish a routine after a time, not all do, so don't compare your baby with any other. As we've said already, the baby who wants frequent feeds will stimulate his mother's breasts and hence her milk supply better than the baby who asks for only five or six feeds a day. If in fact your baby only asks for five feeds a day, be very wary and try giving him more, as five episodes of suckling are not really enough to keep up the milk supply in most women.

How long?

Again, let your baby tell you. The old rule of ten minutes a side was created because that was roughly the average length of time babies seemed to take. Not all babies are average, though, so whereas some of them will need less than ten minutes a side, some will want more. During the first few months you may find that your baby has periods when he wants to feed (or at least to be at the breast) almost continuously for several hours. This is not unusual and is his way of increasing your milk supply. People will tell you that a baby gets most of the milk he needs in the first few minutes at each breast. There is an element of truth in this but studies have shown that not all babies get what they need as quickly. Every baby is different. A lot will depend on how vigorously your baby sucks, the strength of your let-down reflex and the time taken for the let-down to start working. Some babies like to play at the breast and feed sporadically while others go for speed above all else.

Another factor to bear in mind is that some babies enjoy sucking the nipple even if they have emptied the breast. This can be pleasant for you too and there is no reason to stop unless you want to do something else or if you have any soreness of the nipples. This *comfort suckling* is thought by many psychologists to be an important factor in the baby's emotional development. The dummy or thumb are the bottle fed baby's substitutes for comfort suckling at the breast. As your baby gets older, he'll finish his feeds more quickly unless he's tired or upset.

So the answer? There isn't one. When your baby seems to have finished one side – when he becomes less interested in feeding – change him to the other side and let him carry on there as long as he wants to. *Don't watch the clock.* Primitive peoples don't have clocks and they feed their babies more successfully than we do!

One breast or two?

Many babies only drink from one breast during a feed. Provided you alternate the breast you give at each feed and the baby is satisfied, this is fine. Giving both breasts at each feed is a Western idea and is not done in those parts of the world where breast feeding is done more naturally and schedules are unknown. If your baby is extra hungry or fussy, give him both breasts but let him decide. One breast at a time fits in well with the baby who wants frequent small feeds, as many prefer.

Night feeds

The easiest and most natural way of feeding your baby at night is to have him in bed with you all night. This means you'll hardly have to wake up to feed him, because you simply feed him lying down. There'll be no disturbing night-time crying to wake the rest of the household because you can feed him as soon as he becomes restless. And you'll know that he's safe, warm and in the most natural place – next to his parents.

It'll be easier for you not to wear a bra or a nightie at all and in the early weeks this will help prevent any soreness of your nipples by letting the air get to the nipple skin.

Most people are horrified at the suggestion that breast feeding babies should sleep with their parents. Many mothers fear that they'll roll on or suffocate the baby but the chances of doing this are virtually nil. Millions of women the world over sleep with their children quite safely. One of the commonest arguments we hear against this practice is that the baby will become dependent on the mother for sleeping and that he'll be loath to sleep in his own cot or bed when he's older. The way round this is to get the older baby who's stopped breast feeding to sleep in your bed at bedtime and then to transfer him to his own later. Soon he'll get the hang of your new method.

Some mothers feel guilty about having a baby in bed with them. They're uneasy at the thought of prolonged physical contact in bed with their child and some even feel it's incestuous, if the child is a boy. This is obviously nonsense as far as tiny breast feeding babies are concerned.

Should you decide for whatever reason that you don't want to sleep with your baby, make things as easy as you can for yourself at night by keeping the baby's cot near your bed, preferably so close that you don't even have to get out of bed to lift the baby in when he cries. A very little baby will be quite happy in a cot or crib right by your bed. This often isn't easy, though, as most cots are not the right height. If your husband is a do-it-yourself man he will be able to modify the cot to bring the level nearer that of your bed. Hopefully, cot manufacturers will start making them so that the drop side can be lowered to the level of the mother's bed.

Keep nappies by the bed so that they are to hand. Your baby will probably go to sleep quite happily without a nappy change at all after night feeds. 'One-way' nappy liners will help keep his skin dry.

If you can't sleep with the baby in your room at all then either bring him back with you into your bed to feed, where you'll both be warm and comfy, or put on your dressing gown and feed him in his room.

When will your baby stop having night feeds? This again is very much an individual matter. Research suggests that breast fed babies tend to wake more at night. This is scarcely surprising since breast milk is more quickly digested than cows' milk. Your baby may give up his night feeds early, in which case you must make sure that you breast feed often enough during the day to keep up the milk supply and stop your breasts becoming engorged. You may have to express some milk before you go to bed or even during the night to prevent discomfort. Some mothers wake their babies for a feed before they go to bed if they have given up night feeds too early and the milk supply seems to be dwindling. On the other hand your baby may want to continue with one, two or even more night feeds for many months. If your baby wants feeding more often than once or twice your husband may help by getting up for you and bringing the baby to you in bed, then putting him back into his cot after the feed. Babies often want frequent feeds when they're very young and occasionally for the odd night or two when they are older, so it's worth accepting and coping with them as best you can. Broken nights will make you tired, so you'll have to try and catch up on your sleep during the day. Your relaxation practice at ante-natal classes may come in useful here. One consolation for the breast feeding mother is that bottle fed babies often take much longer to settle after a night feed than breast fed babies do.

Many mothers notice during the first few weeks of breast feeding particularly that when their breasts are full, they feel hot and may sweat suddenly. This is especially likely to happen at night. It is a helpful signal that the time has come to feed your baby – the longer full breasts are left unemptied, the more likely they are to become engorged – so wake your baby up.

Leaking

The leaking you'll have noticed during the first few weeks may gradually become less of a problem. This is partly because the let-down reflex becomes more controlled as your milk supply becomes established, and partly because the storage capacity of the milk ducts increases during the first few weeks so that they can hold the let-down milk without allowing it to escape. You'll still notice leaking from the opposite breast during a feed though.

How you'll feel at different times

As milk is secreted constantly by the milk-producing cells of the breasts, the amount of milk in the breast will depend to some extent on the length of time since the last feed. You'll soon learn to judge when your baby might ask for a feed because your breasts will feel full and may even leak. If your baby doesn't wake and your breasts are uncomfortable, either express some milk or wake the baby up – after all, *you need him* sometimes to relieve you as much as he needs you at other times to relieve his hunger.

As your baby will hopefully have his longest break between

feeds at night, you'll notice this fullness in your breasts first thing in the morning especially. You may even wake up with your nightie and sheets drenched with milk. The early morning feed is often the most pleasant simply because of the very real sense of relief you get.

During the day the enjoyment you get from feeding will depend to some extent on how busy you are. If feeds are slotted into a packed day, you probably won't feel very calm and the baby may sense your tension and be more fussy than usual. Be careful not to be so tense that your let-down doesn't work. If you don't experience the tell-tale signs (see page 100) then do your best to slow down a bit for the rest of the day and cut out a few jobs the next day. Many mothers feel at their worst in the early evening. Not only do they have to feed the other children and start getting them to bed but they also want to tidy up the house, feed the baby, and start thinking about supper. It may all be just too much for your milk supply so try and organize things so they don't all happen at once. Your husband's supper can wait, as long as he understands why and has something to eat to keep him going in the meantime; the other children must learn how to clear up their own toys; and you could give them their tea earlier. Do anything to avoid having lots of things to do at the very time of the day when you're beginning to feel tired anyway. Prepare food for the evening in the afternoon, make full use of your refrigerator and freezer and do dishes like casseroles that can be prepared in advance.

Crying

The sound of your baby's cry is designed to alert you so that you tend him. It's not the sort of sound that can easily be ignored, even by a stranger, and a baby that won't stop crying is very disturbing. If a baby seems to do nothing but cry for the first few weeks or even months, it's hardly surprising that so many mothers feel something must be wrong with the baby or its food. Once they are reassured by the doctor or health visitor that nothing is wrong with the baby, the next step is often to change the food, and for a breast feeding mother this means giving the baby a bottle of cows' milk.

Is this necessary? In almost every case the answer is no. The first thing to do is to breast feed properly, in the way Nature intended, which means at least every time the baby cries. A baby breast fed on schedule will almost certainly cry a lot because not only is he hungry before the clock says it is time for his next feed but he is also denied comfort suckling time because his mother thinks she must only allow him ten minutes on each breast. Feeding a baby when he cries, for as long as he wants to feed, will almost certainly reduce the amount of crying he does. It will also increase your milk supply, which is a good thing if he was crying because he was hungry. Research has shown that breast fed babies fed on demand cry much less than schedule breast fed babies. The psychological effects of long periods of crying are difficult to evaluate but not difficult to guess at.

Some babies crave company and will only settle when they are held. One way to cope with this if there are things you have to do is to buy a baby sling. There are several on the market which will leave your hands free to get on with your work but which will keep the baby securely next to you as you walk around.

Other babies can be pacified (as long as they are not hungry) by a ride in their pram or in a car. Anything is worth trying but always try comfort suckling first.

If all else fails, ask a relative or neighbour to look after the baby for a time to give you a break. If you are constantly worried about the crying, your milk supply will dwindle and that will make your baby cry more. A change of face and scene often quietens a baby miraculously.

Bowels

A totally breast fed baby's motions are not foul-smelling like those of a bottle fed baby. They are passed very frequently at first but later may be passed only every few days. Their normal colour is a bright yellow. Often your baby will open his bowels during a feed, so you'll find it saves washing if you change his nappy after a feed, unless he is one of those babies who won't feed in a wet nappy.

Some everyday 'problems'

The mother in the house on her own will come up against some practical problems when she is feeding her baby. For instance, what does she do if the doorbell rings? There are four ways round this. You can decide that when you are feeding, nothing is going to stop you, so you don't answer the bell. You can do up your clothes quickly and answer the door either with your hungry baby crying in your arms or left safely somewhere. You can carry on feeding and answer the door anyway, perhaps with a shawl round you. Or you can make a little notice for the front door which says 'I am feeding my baby. Only ring if it is important, please.'

What about the window cleaner? That's easier. Always keep a nappy or shawl near you when you are feeding so that you can do a cover-up job to preserve your modesty! Practise first so that you learn how to do it without annoying the baby.

The telephone is more difficult because somehow it always seems such an urgent noise and it's difficult to steel yourself to leave it unanswered. One way round this is to take the phone off the hook while you're feeding. Another is to have the phone by you. This may need organizing with the GPO who can put the phone anywhere you want provided you pay for the alteration.

With any of these disturbances, what you don't want to happen is for your let-down to be inhibited and for the feed to be spoilt, so it's worth thinking about how you are going to cope before you actually have to. Your let-down will work best when you are calm and undisturbed.

Feeding with the children around

A new baby in the family is both a joy and a misery to the other children, especially if they are very young themselves. The attractions of the new acquisition are tempered by the fact that mother now has a new central interest in her life which seems to take up most of her time.

The way round this is to be extra loving, especially to your youngest child, because it is he who will be most affected by the new baby. If he wants to have a feed – let him – he's only trying to compete for your attention and will soon get fed up with the breast.

Always try to bring your older children into the breast feeding circle if they're interested. Soon you'll be so adept at breast feeding you'll be able to sit reading to a toddler and breast feeding the baby at the same time. If you find you can't do this then keep an absorbing toy or game handy for feed times or reserve a few minutes to play alone later with the child who feels left out.

How to feed in company

Again, there are many ways of coping with this and what you decide to do will depend on you and your feelings of modesty and on the people involved. You may discover that you always prefer to feed alone, in which case you'll miss hours of other people's company. If you do decide on this, then you can either send visitors into another room when you feed in the room you usually use or you can go into another room yourself. You and the baby are just as important as the visitors. Don't hurry the feed in order to get back to your friends and show off the baby. The baby will be much more likely to be in a good mood for being shown off if he's well fed and happy and that means feeding him as you normally would.

If you are in someone else's house, make yourself warm and comfortable before you feed and ask for drinks or cushions or whatever you need.

If you are happy to feed in company you might like a few tips. Some people are embarrassed about seeing a baby being breast fed simply because they are not used to it. If you sense these feelings, your let-down might not work. You can get round this either by sitting at one end of a room so that you can join in the discussion but not be too boldly in evidence, or by draping yourself with a shawl to cover both breast and baby. Of course some people are delighted to see a baby fed naturally and are not at all embarrassed.

Shawl draping is useful when you are in a train, bus, park or eating out – all occasions when other people may be embarrassed even though you're not.

Entertaining

If looking after people and cooking for them comes easily to you, then you'll probably find breast feeding no hindrance to entertaining. However, if you're the sort of person who worries for days about what to give friends to eat, then don't entertain for the months you're feeding your baby. It's as simple as that. Whatever you cook, make sure it's something that won't be harmed by being left in a warm oven if you have to feed the baby before you eat. The calmer you are, the calmer the baby will be as babies quickly pick up their mothers' feelings and react to them.

Car journeys and holidays

Breast feeding is easy in a car – in fact it really comes into its own when you're travelling. Either stop and feed or carry on (with your husband driving, of course!) and feed the baby in the back seat for safety. You should have no problem at all.

If you are going to fly, it's not a bad idea to fly at night so that the baby will be sleepy, the aircraft dark for feeding and the chances of your having more privacy increased because fewer passengers move about. Some airlines have a special seat that can be curtained off for the breast feeding mother, but really the answer is for her to feed discreetly in the main part of the aircraft.

When you're travelling, don't get exhausted. Let your husband do as much as possible or you could impair your let-down reflex temporarily.

Holidays are much simpler with a breast fed baby. There's no sterilizing to worry about, no boiled water to organize for a feed and the equipment necessary is always to hand.

Going out

Whenever you go out, try to take your baby with you. Once your baby has become used to you being there all the time a bottle (even of breast milk) may not comfort him. What he needs is his mother.

If you have to go out without your baby then you'll either have to leave a bottle of cows' milk or express some of your own milk and leave that instead. Many mothers will be loath to leave even an occasional bottle of cows' milk after our discussion about cows' milk in chapter 3. This is sensible in the first four months or so, but probably doesn't matter after that. In the first four months, expressed breast milk can be left in the fridge in a sterile bottle and the bottle warmed up in a bowl of hot water when needed by your baby sitter. If the baby is hungry enough he'll drink from the bottle and because the milk is his usual brew, there should be no fuss. If he's reluctant to drink from the bottle, then leave instructions with your sitter to give the milk from a sterilized spoon.

We have already described the technique of expressing milk (see page 96). The difficulty is when to do it so as to collect enough. Try expressing after every feed for two days before you are due to go out. In this way you should get enough milk to make up a whole feed. The milk can be expressed directly into a bottle and kept in the fridge for up to three days. You'll notice that the milk goes into layers on standing but these soon disappear when it is warmed.

It's obviously easier to take the baby with you wherever you go and apart from going to the theatre, cinema, a restaurant or a few other places, it should almost always be possible.

Weight gain and clinic attendance

So long as your baby is obviously thriving and happy and has a wet nappy at every feed, then the actual weight gained is of little importance and there is no need to have him weighed frequently, if at all. Remember that many weight charts are based on the average *bottle* fed baby's weight, which is almost certainly too high.

If you do have your baby weighed regularly, don't take any notice of the change from one week to another. Even a healthy, thriving baby sometimes gains no weight or may even lose some in any one week, though the overall rate of gain over the weeks is steady.

If the weight gain is small or non-existent over a few weeks, don't be put off breast feeding but ask your doctor for help to increase your milk supply. If your doctor or health visitor immediately advise complementary feeds, take their advice with a pinch of salt and ring your National Childbirth Trust Breast Feeding Counsellor for her help in increasing your milk supply. If you know how, you can do it by yourself anyway within forty-eight hours. (See page 129) You may also have a La Leche League group near you in which case you can ask their group leader for help. A fully breast fed baby *can* be underfed, especially with our Western 'token' breast feeding, so don't be lulled into complacency. However, in almost every case the milk supply can be increased to meet the baby's needs.

If you have any reason to worry about your baby's health, you must of course see your doctor. It's worth carrying on with breast feeding whatever happens, because even if your baby has cows' milk complements, he'll still do better if he has some breast milk.

Going to the clinic is helpful in that it gives you a chance to discuss things with your health visitor and have your baby's developmental progress checked at intervals by the clinic doctor. You'll also meet other mothers with little children and so strike up some friendships.

We would hasten to add here that we're not decrying baby clinics. They serve a very useful purpose and often ensure that children who are not doing well are channelled to expert help.

What does concern us, though, is that so many of the professional staff employed in baby clinics are not geared to giving good advice about breast feeding. Their training is more likely to have concentrated on the bottle fed baby. So unless a mother sails through breast feeding by herself she may well not find them very helpful when it comes to problems.

Feeding a baby from day to day is one of the most rewarding things in a woman's life, yet may not be as easy as she thinks, unless she is lucky. Knowing what to do is half the battle. Knowing what can go wrong is the other.

9 Looking after yourself

There are two very good reasons for looking after yourself when you've had a baby. Firstly, as wife and mother you're probably the kingpin of your home and if you are well and happy the chances are that the rest of the family will be happy too. If, like so many mothers, you get tired and run down with the pressures of house, husband, other children and baby to look after, then your mood will reflect on the other people in the house.

Secondly, a fit and healthy mother is far more likely to breast feed her baby successfully than the mother who is permanently physically and emotionally exhausted. This is not so much because the amount of milk produced will be greater – we don't know whether this is so or not – and certainly the quality of the milk will be no different, but is because an exhausted mother's let-down reflex just won't be as reliable. Once the let-down reflex becomes unreliable, the baby gets frustrated at each feed and is likely to take less and less milk, become hungry, cry more and so add to the mother's exhaustion.

As we've already described, 'mothering the mother' is seen as a vital part of successful child-rearing in many cultures. These wise people know that a well-cared-for mother stands more chance of rearing her young children happily. In our culture, it's unlikely that you will have somebody to look after you all the time, even if you manage to arrange for a helper to come in for part of the day, so you must make sure that you look after yourself and make this one of your priorities for everyone's sake.

Rest, relaxation and sleep

If you have only one baby, you'll find it comparatively easy to make time for catnaps during the day when the baby sleeps.

Indeed, if you are waking up several times a night, which is highly likely at first, you *must* make time for naps, even if you are the sort of person who would have turned her nose up at daytime sleeping before you had the baby.

For the mother who comes home after forty-eight hours in hospital, rest – and that means rest in bed – is *not* a luxury, it's a must. It's a pretty safe rule to say that you should aim to be spending most of your day in and around your bed for the first eight days after the birth whether you're in hospital or at home. This doesn't mean you should stay in bed *all day* – you shouldn't. But you certainly shouldn't be busying yourself around the house.

The temptation, especially for the efficient sort of woman who held down a job before she had her baby, is to cram all sorts of household and other tasks into the baby's sleep time. As we've said before, you have the rest of your life to be a superwoman – you don't have to be one now. If you can be rested, cheerful and happy, you'll be a far better mother than if you'd cleaned the oven, changed the sheets, written ten letters and exhausted yourself! Keep your kitchen and bathroom clean, pick up obvious fluff and tidy up things left lying around – that's all you need to do to give the illusion of a spotless home. Housework is always there – you'll probably only have a chance to mother a new baby a couple of times in a lifetime – make the most of them.

Whenever you can, then, relax. Even if you don't sleep during the day, lie down on your bed and read or put the radio on. Think about moving the TV into the bedroom. Use your relaxation training from ante-natal classes so that every muscle is relaxed. You can even do this when you're feeding the baby, peeling the vegetables, watching television or driving the car. The secret is not to let muscle tension build up.

Demand feeding is Nature's way of ensuring that newly delivered mothers sit down quietly in the days immediately after birth.

At night you'll just need to accept the fact that it'll be a long time before you regularly have a long, unbroken stretch of sleep. If you go back to sleep quickly when you've fed the baby, so much the better. If you can't, don't worry, just relax. At least you'll be getting physical rest. If you keep your baby in bed with you, you'll hardly lose any sleep anyway.

The mother with more than one child has a much harder task if she is to get enough rest. If the elder child still sleeps during the day, then she should make every effort to feed the baby before the toddler goes for his sleep, so she can have a rest at the same time. If this is impossible, then it's a good idea to lie down anyway and feed the baby in bed – that's always more relaxing than sitting in a chair. Sometimes you'll be able to get a neighbour or a friend to help by taking the toddler off your hands for an hour while you sleep. He'll probably like the change too. An extension of this is to get a group of young local mothers together so that you can help each other out when you've got baby problems.

The food you eat

There is no evidence that any food, drink or vitamins will increase or decrease your milk supply (see chapter 10) providing you eat a well-balanced nutritious diet. It's sensible to eat according to your appetite and not to try and lose weight – the fat stores you will have accumulated during pregnancy will slowly be lost with breast feeding as long as you are not overeating. The mother who eats sensibly will not only provide her baby with plenty of milk but will also make sure that her own body isn't drained of food resources for the baby's sake.

Even severely malnourished mothers in underdeveloped countries manage to feed their babies for three months before extra food is necessary for the normal growth of the baby. However, they often do this at the expense of their own bodies – they can become short of calcium and protein, for example. The more babies these women have and feed, the poorer their physical state becomes. We must stress, though, that this situation is virtually never seen in the affluent West where almost everyone has enough to eat.

What would happen if you didn't eat enough? There's a chance that you might not produce as much milk as you could and that your baby might go hungry. The actual quality of your milk would be relatively little affected. Obviously you can't go on a slimming spree while you're feeding.

How much extra should you eat? This is a vexed question that experts have been discussing for years. Recommended extra calorie allowances change every few years in the light of more up-to-date knowledge. What we can say, though, is that you should eat slightly more than you do when you are not pregnant or breast feeding (that is if you usually eat normally). Given that the baby needs an average (depending on size) of between 600 and 800 calories daily from you and given that your accumulated fat stores built up during pregnancy should supply 300 calories daily to the milk, then it would seem that you should be eating an extra 300–500 calories a day. Some experts have found, though, that mothers breast feeding successfully eat on average almost 700 calories a day more than bottle feeding mothers and still manage to lose weight!

Is there anything you should eat more of when you are feeding your baby? No. Assuming you're eating a good diet, just eat slightly more of everything and you'll be all right.

Provided your diet is well-balanced, there's absolutely no need to drink a lot of milk. Indeed, if you don't like milk there's no need to drink any at all! Cows' milk doesn't make breast milk. Calcium can be absorbed from several other foods besides dairy products (see page 81), so don't worry.

You'll find, though, that you are more thirsty than usual and this is scarcely surprising when you consider that the baby will be taking on average between 600 and 800 ml (more than a pint) of milk a day from you, depending on the individual baby, his age and weight. There is no need to force yourself to drink more – just drink as much as you want to. Research has shown that drinking more than your thirst demands actually reduces the amount of milk you produce.

Many nursing mothers feel most thirsty while they are actually feeding, so keep something by you then.

Many mothers worry whether or not they should drink anything alcoholic. Drinking in moderation is quite acceptable and won't hurt you or your baby. Some alcohol will pass into your breast milk and of course if you drink large amounts, correspondingly more will get to the baby. There is a report of an eight-day-old baby who became drunk after the mother had had 750 ml (well over a pint) of port in a period of twenty-four hours! Drinking enough to make you feel 'tipsy' will harm your milk supply by effecting oxytocin output. So go easy!

Some spicy foods like garlic and curry can come through in the milk but as far as we know they have no effect on the baby. The vast majority of foods don't get through to your milk, so don't worry. There are no foods that are absolutely forbidden but should you find that your baby reacts in an unusual way to breast milk after you have eaten something different, then cut it out while you're breast feeding.

Smoking may reduce your milk supply and the nicotine will pass to the baby in the milk. As nicotine in large enough amounts has unpleasant side-effects, it's a good idea to cut out smoking completely if you can and at any rate to cut down the number of cigarettes you smoke while you're breast feeding.

Contraception

Unless you're keen to have another baby soon, you'll need to take contraceptive precautions even if you're fully breast feeding. Although, as we've seen on page 62 you won't ovulate for some time, breast feeding can't be relied upon as a 100 per cent safe contraceptive.

As the various contraceptive pills are unsuitable (see page 129) this means you will have to use some sort of barrier method or, later, an intra-uterine contraceptive device. Probably the safest and most satisfactory contraceptives to use soon after a baby are diaphragms and sheaths. A diaphragm should be fitted at a Family Planning Clinic or by your doctor and should then be used with a spermicidal cream. A sheath for your husband may be the most practical and satisfactory method overall until you stop breast feeding and go back on to the pill (if you were on it before) or have an IUCD fitted.

Going out (see also page 116)
If you and your husband go out to friends for the evening, then take the baby with you, even if you have a sitter for the older children. If the baby wants feeding, it's a simple enough matter to pop upstairs and feed and if your hostess has been warned in advance that you are bringing your breast fed baby, she won't have cooked anything that might spoil if left in the oven for an extra hour.

Shopping
If you normally travel some way to the shops you'll find in the early weeks that you will have very little time between feeds to do the shopping. You can get round this by doing a big weekly shop with your husband and the car or by getting the shops to deliver. Some mothers still have corner shops near them. There's nothing worse, though, than going shopping and having to wheel a starving, crying baby home in a laden pram.

One last word. Don't expect to get back to feeling like your old self overnight. Having a baby is physically and emotionally very demanding and many women don't feel like their real selves for the first month. Many women say that it takes a full year to get back to normal physically and mentally.

10 Your milk supply

Whilst many mothers never have any problems at all with supplying the right amount of milk for their babies, others find that they have too much or too little, especially in the early weeks before their milk supply has become properly established. Too much milk is often a nuisance but rarely stops a mother from breast feeding. Too little milk, however, is the commonest reason mothers give for stopping breast feeding or for introducing complementary feeds in the first few weeks.

Research has shown that women who *really* want to breast feed actually produce more milk than those who don't want to or who are apathetic about it.

Studies show that between 40 and 72 per cent of mothers who start breast feeding fully in hospital but stop in the first two weeks, stop because they think (or they are told) that they have insufficient milk. It's interesting to look further at these two figures. The first comes from a survey in Aberdeen in 1951–3. The hospital concerned made a point of test weighing babies to assess the adequacy of their mothers' milk production in the first few days – hardly a procedure likely to instil confidence into a nursing mother! The second figure comes from a survey in Nottingham in 1957. Further questioning of these mothers revealed that 55 per cent of them had not wanted to breast feed anyway, so in fact the actual number stopping because of inadequate milk was smaller than would seem. The reason was simply used as an 'excuse' for stopping.

But having said this, the fact remains that a lot of women who really want to breast feed fail because they believe they haven't enough milk. Many a woman's greatest single concern *before* she embarks on breast feeding is that she won't have enough milk. The worry seems to be ingrained in modern women.

In practice, almost every woman can breast feed if she wants to and if she is given enough information and help to back her up. Experiments in which women who said they hadn't enough milk were given oxytocin injections after a feed showed that in the majority about 50 per cent of the available milk was still in the breast. Because their let-down reflex (Nature's own oxytocin supply) hadn't worked, this 50 per cent was trapped in the breast and wasn't available for the baby. Almost every woman can supply about twice the volume of milk her baby needs to thrive. The trouble is that she doesn't always let it down to her baby. Your milk supply *can* be increased – it's simply a question of knowing how.

Is your baby getting enough?

This is a loaded question – the very fact that it's asked at all is enough to worry many mothers so much that their milk production falls off and their babies don't in fact get enough!

It's a question that stems from the years when strict four-hourly schedules were enforced, when many babies really *didn't* get enough because the schedules didn't allow milk production to reach its full potential.

It's also a question that would rarely need to be asked at all if only mothers were encouraged to breast feed as Nature intended.

However, as so many mothers today are still wrongly advised to restrict suckling time to some sort of schedule or routine, it's a question that must be asked.

If a baby is alert, happy, satisfied after a feed and obviously thriving, then he's getting enough. An underfed baby is often very placid, though he may cry unduly and not appear to be satisfied after a feed. The average thriving baby gains weight at a rate of approximately four to seven ounces a week, though this gain need not be a regular one every week. Many healthy babies gain less than this on a regular basis. Whatever you do, don't use any baby scales at home. The neurotic weighing of your baby at home is a sure way to get yourself into a real panic as soon as his weight gain doesn't live up to your unrealistic expectations. Remember too that the so-called 'normal' weights are often based on bottle-fed (on average overweight) babies. If your baby consistently lags a little behind yet is well and happy, don't worry. Research has shown that we are foolish to judge how healthy a baby is by his weight gain in the early months. A study in southern Africa has found that in communities in which babies gain weight and grow quickly, the population as a whole tends to die younger. Early growth goes hand in hand with early senescence.

An underfed baby will not soak as many nappies as a well-fed one. This is difficult to assess, though, as the nappies of a schedule-fed baby will probably be changed less often and so will be quite likely to be very wet anyway. Similarly, an underfed baby will not dirty the nappy as much but this is an unreliable way of deciding whether your baby is getting enough.

If you or a professional adviser think that your baby is not getting enough, for whatever reason, then you must take steps to increase your milk supply. Before we talk about how to do this, though, let's just run through the factors that affect milk supply.

Factors affecting milk supply

1 *Mother's age*. Older mothers having their first babies tend to produce less milk at first than younger ones. This particularly applies to women over thirty. It does not mean that their milk supply cannot be increased.

2 *Mother's attitude*. Mothers who *really* want to breast feed actually produce more milk. One study of mothers' attitudes to feeding their babies found that those who had said they preferred bottle feeding were three times more likely to say that their baby had refused the breast and twice as likely to say that their baby was a bad feeder, when compared with mothers whose intention it was to breast feed right from the start. Breast feeding is thus greatly helped by positive attitudes. In the same survey, mothers who wanted to breast feed reported that their babies refused the bottle!

3 *Mother's parity*. Mothers having their first babies tend to produce less milk than those who already have one or more

babies. Again, this is not to say that their milk supply cannot be increased.

4 *Suckling.* We've already seen in chapter 2 that the more you suckle your baby, the more prolactin is secreted by the pituitary gland, the more milk is produced by the breasts and the better conditioned the let-down reflex becomes. It's the total length of suckling time each day that is important and that depends on the number and length of the feeds, together with the time given to comfort suckling (see page 108). Your baby will ask for a certain number of feeds, which you should always give. He may also want to carry on feeding when the milk is finished; you should allow as much of this as you can. You may also have to offer a certain number of unasked-for feeds in order to build up your supply if he's not getting enough.

5 *The let-down reflex.* Even if you allow your baby plenty of suckling time, there's a chance that your let-down reflex may not work, in which case the baby will only get the foremilk. Let-down failure is a very common cause of insufficient milk. The let-down reflex must work if the baby is to get the hindmilk and so empty the breast. If your let-down usually takes two to three minutes to work and you normally restrict suckling time to say ten minutes, your baby will have lost two to three minutes of what you thought was 'drinking time'. While seven to eight minutes' drinking time is enough for some babies, it'll leave others very hungry indeed.

6 *The degree of emptying of the breast.* This is tied up with the last two points. If your baby isn't allowed long enough to empty the breast, if the hindmilk isn't let down, or if the breast is allowed to remain full for a long period before the baby feeds, then the milk supply will gradually fall off. This is because the tension in the breast from the build-up of milk reduces the blood supply in the milk glands, so making the milk-producing cells less efficient. Secondly, the tension actually harms the milk-producing cells, so making them less able to produce milk. Thirdly, the muscle cells cannot contract so well round the swollen milk glands and so the let-down is less efficient.

Whenever your breasts feel full or the slightest bit tense and uncomfortable, you should give your baby a feed.

7 *Diet.* Providing you eat well your diet should make no difference to your milk supply, bearing in mind that you should be eating slightly more than normal and drinking according to your thirst. Malnourished women produce less milk, though the quality of their milk is little affected.

8 *The pill.* The contraceptive pill, unless it is of the progestogen-only type, usually reduces the milk supply.

How to increase your milk supply

There are two ways of doing this. The first is to increase suckling time, that is the number and length of feeds, and the second is to improve the let-down reflex, if this is at fault.

1 *Suckling time.* Breast feeding as commonly practised in the West today is really a sort of 'token' effort. It is governed by schedules and the restriction of suckling time and usually lasts only for a few weeks, during which time cows' milk, juices or solids are added to the baby's diet.

Natural breast feeding depends on the supply and demand principle, which ensures that the breasts automatically produce enough milk for the individual baby. There is no limitation of suckling time and no need for any food supplements for the first four to six months at least.

The first thing to do when increasing suckling time is to *feed your baby when he is hungry*. How do you know when he is hungry? The answer is, when he cries.

You may already be feeding your baby when he 'asks' and yet still not have enough milk for him, in which case there are two things you can do. *Firstly, let your baby feed as long as he wants on each breast.* Secondly, *fit in some extra feeds*, even if your baby doesn't actually ask for them. This may mean waking him up but as it's for his own good (and yours), do it anyway.

If you increase your baby's suckling time by building up the number and length of his feeds, then your milk supply will improve because of the greater secretion of prolactin, the conditioning of the let-down reflex and the better and more frequent emptying of the breasts. This usually takes at least two days.

2 *The let-down reflex.* As we explained in chapter 2, the let-down reflex is readily influenced by such factors as fatigue, anxiety, fear and pain, so much so that these factors can completely prevent the let-down of milk. During the first few weeks or months the let-down is more vulnerable than later when the milk supply has become established and the nursing mother is more confident in her ability to feed her baby. This goes part of the way towards explaining why a mother nursing her second baby is more successful from the start than when she nursed her first.

When we talk about the establishment of the milk supply, we mean that the let-down reflex has become so well-conditioned through practice that it virtually never fails and also that the mother's breasts are matching their milk supply to the baby's demands, with no surplus or shortage.

Poor milk supply due to an unreliable let-down reflex is one of the commonest problems of breast feeding but once you understand what is happening, there's every chance of putting it right. Successful breast feeding depends more on good drainage of the milk that is produced (which of course depends on the proper working of the let-down reflex) – than on the actual amount that is produced. The vast majority of women can produce more than enough milk – the successful breast feeders are those who can release this milk from their breasts.

How do you know if your let-down reflex is working?

In the early days you'll know by the afterpains in the womb early in a feed and by a tingling feeling in the breasts together with spraying or leaking of milk from the nipples. The skin of the breasts feels warmer than usual and any initial nipple pain disappears as the milk floods through, so equalizing the negative pressure created by the baby sucking. Having said this, some women experience none of these sensations yet have perfectly good let-down reflexes.

How can you make sure that your let-down reflex works properly and reliably?

Check through the following points:

1 Be calm, unhurried, and enjoy the feeds. Have everything you need (for you, the baby and other children) to hand.

Decide in advance what you will do about the phone, the front door bell, the window cleaner and other people who may be with you in the room (see page 114).

Cut out things which worry you but are inessential, such as unnecessary entertaining, letter writing, telephoning, cooking gourmet meals and so on.

Cut down on other activities so that you always have time for feeds and are never in a hurry to do something else. This will mean that you don't give promises to be anywhere at any set time but explain that you'll come when you're ready. Exceptions to this may have to be visits to the clinic, your doctor and so on.

Relax both before and during a feed by going through your relaxation technique learnt at ante-natal classes and by trying to clear your mind of any worries. While this sounds difficult, it'll come with practice.

2 Keep yourself fit. Make sure you are eating and drinking sensibly. (See page 121.)

Don't get overtired – have several naps during the day if possible; put your feet up whenever you sit down; don't do unnecessary housework and other chores; organize shopping in the easiest way possible and cut down on outside commitments for a while.

3 Condition your let-down reflex. Try and get into a routine before a feed – a regular chain of events will condition your let-down into working reliably.

Don't be tempted to skip night feeds – you need them as much as the baby does.

When your breasts feel tense and full, wake the baby for a feed – try not to let him sleep for long periods – your breasts need regular emptying.

If your milk lets down unexpectedly, wake your baby and feed him.

4 *Other points.* Make sure you're comfortable when feeding – aching shoulders or a draught round your feet won't help.

If you have sore nipples, try and get your let-down to work before the baby feeds. Remember that the pain will soon go and certainly won't last throughout a feed. (See page 143.)

A nasal spray containing synthetic oxytocin (Syntocinon) is available on prescription and will help your let-down if all else fails. Use this to give yourself confidence that you've got plenty of milk and then stop using it.

Have a small alcoholic drink just before a feed – this will relax you and help your let-down. (But see page 123.)

Some mothers find a hot shower helps their let-down though this obviously isn't practical before every feed. You can even feed in the bath.

There are several pitfalls to avoid when breast feeding, things which you can't know about beforehand unless you've read a lot about breast feeding and which may make you think your milk supply is poor. Unfortunately, your professional advisers may not know about them either and may therefore give you misleading or frankly wrong advice.

One of the commonest reasons that women think they have insufficient milk is that they expect their babies to take exactly the same amount of milk at each feed. Should the baby want more than his mother can supply at one particular feed, she worries because she thinks she'll never be able to make enough milk for him again.

However, babies don't necessarily want the same amount to eat from feed to feed let alone from day to day. Your milk supply won't necessarily match up with your baby's increased appetite, so be prepared that on some days your baby may be hungry. This happens to almost every mother and baby from time to time but is rarely mentioned in feeding manuals written for either mothers or professionals.

If your baby has previously been well satisfied with your milk but suddenly becomes edgy and miserable and you think he is still hungry after a feed, you must increase your milk supply to match his increased needs. If you're already feeding on demand, give him a couple of extra feeds during the day, or even more if you have time. The increased nipple stimulation will soon increase your milk production, though it will be a day or two before supply catches up with demand.

Another pitfall is that when you return home from hospital, whether it's at two or ten days, your milk supply is likely to dwindle temporarily because of the change, the excitement and the extra work you may find yourself doing. Family doctors say that they frequently receive calls from mothers just home saying that their milk has gone. Of course it hasn't and they can increase it – there's no need to give the baby a bottle or stop breast feeding because there is a temporary decrease in supply. If you realize the problem may crop up, you'll probably be able to cope better. Follow the advice on page 119 and your milk won't dry up.

Cows' milk complements

If you were persuaded to let your baby have cows' milk as well as breast milk in hospital, don't worry – it's quite possible to start breast feeding fully once you get home.

Reduce the amount of cows' milk in the bottle by about half an ounce at each feed, so your baby will want more breast milk each time.

After two days of increased suckling time, letting the baby suck as much as he wants to even on an empty breast, your milk supply will begin to increase. Be prepared for two days of very frequent feeding – perhaps as much as forty minutes every two hours. Look after yourself by doing as few other things as possible – just rest and cuddle the baby. It's perfectly possible to build up your milk supply if you have the confidence and patience to do it.

What if all should fail

If you've got this far in the book you'll have read enough to be thoroughly disappointed if you do fail at breast feeding. Unfortunately, with the best will in the world a few women will be genetically unable to breast feed possibly because over many generations babies of their forebears who were poor breast feeders were kept alive by wet nurses and bottle feeding whereas if left to Nature they would have died. Should you be one of these, don't despair – it's not the end of the world! After all, there is an alternative and such breast feeding as you have been able to do will have been better than nothing. The important thing is not to transfer your disappointment to your baby – it's certainly not his fault and it probably isn't yours either. Your attachment to and love for your child are more important than your milk.

Before you give up completely, though, give the complementary feeds with a spoon, not a bottle. You may find that you'll have enough milk to give him the occasional feed – perhaps in the early morning. What's more, with the relief of your anxiety over starving him, your let-down might start working well.

We suggest using a spoon for complementary feeds because once your baby has become used to the different technique of drinking from a bottle, he'll be very loath to accept your nipple. Studies have shown that levels of breast feeding can be raised by 50 per cent in hospitals allowing complementary feeds to be given only by spoon.

If it comes to the crunch, a loving, caring mother is what a baby really needs most so don't let things get so on top of you that you ruin your unique relationship. When you feed him with a bottle, hold him exactly as you did when breast feeding and don't suddenly treat him like a doll – held at arm's length.

If you ever have another baby, try again. You'll be a lot more confident as a mother and will have experience that is bound to help. Failure to breast feed the first time simply means that you will need more help and back-up the next time. It's up to you to make sure you get it. Contact the National Childbirth Trust or La Leche League for help well before the time comes.

Is your baby getting too much?

In the early days, before your milk supply has become established so that it matches your baby's demands, you may have too much milk for him. Over the days the supply will gradually adjust but the abundance can cause some problems, especially towards the end of the first week. A newborn baby can be bewildered and almost choked by an over-exuberant flow of milk. He'll turn his head away, cough and splutter and be reluctant to go on feeding. He will also swallow too much air as he tries to drink from this 'fire hydrant' and this can produce colic – rarely seen in breast fed babies.

You can cope with this by expressing some milk before a feed, either by hand or by letting the milk leak away if your let-down works before your baby is put to the breast.

If you allow your breasts to become overfull by letting your baby sleep too long between feeds, the same problem can arise. Wake him when your breasts feel full and tense, otherwise he'll be overwhelmed by the flow later.

As your baby grows, he'll be better able to cope with an efficient, fast let-down reflex without choking. You should think yourself lucky if this is your 'problem' – better to have a good let-down than an unreliable, weak one.

If you and the clinic think that your wholly breast fed baby is too fat, then you can cut down your milk production gradually by reducing the number and length of feeds. The idea that breast fed babies never get fat is of course wrong – some do – and it's worth while doing something about it sooner rather than later.

If you always have too much milk for your baby, think about donating the extra to a milk bank, where it would be used for premature babies whose mothers didn't want to or couldn't breast feed. Ask your doctor or health visitor how to go about this in your area.

Old wives' tales abound on the subject of increasing milk supply and it's probably fair to say that when there are lots of conflicting old wives' tales, none is any good. There's no harm in following them, though, provided you also carry out our proven methods above. The danger comes when mothers rely solely on these fairy tale methods of feeding successfully and forget the basic principles. Because you know someone for whom these old remedies worked, it doesn't mean that they'll work for you. By the time you've worked through even a small proportion of all the available 'cures', your milk will be gone for good.

Some you'll doubtless be given are that Vitamin B will work wonders – in fact its only benefit will possibly be to make you feel well in yourself, though that may help indirectly; that alcohol, especially heavy beers, will help – again they may (in small amounts only), but only by making you relaxed and so aiding your let-down reflex; that vitamin E will increase your milk supply – there's no scientific proof of this; that drinking cows' milk will make more breast milk – quite wrong; that drinking more fluid than you actually need will make more milk – in fact it can do the opposite, the secret is to drink what you want; and that there are magic drugs which will increase your milk supply.

Chlorpromazine, other phenothiazine drugs and the rauwolfia group of drugs do increase the milk supply but they should be used very much as a last resort, if at all. A new approach to stimulating the milk supply with drugs involves the use of metoclopramide, a drug normally used for gastric troubles which was found to stimulate the secretion of prolactin. Small trials have shown that this really does increase the milk supply but as with all drugs we have to ask ourselves what else it might be doing as well.

Adequacy of milk is not solely a concern of Western women – throughout the centuries women in many cultures have used amulets, potions, herbal skin rubs, chants and prayers to ensure they will have the right amount of milk. With our present knowledge of breast feeding we know that these methods are unnecessary. By following the simple rules outlined above we can ensure that we will have enough milk for our babies without recourse to any magic. Indeed, moral support and reassurance are often all that are needed.

11 The working mother

When we talk to mothers about their reasons for *not* breast feeding it isn't long before the subject of getting back to work crops up. Women have now become an important part of the work force in the Western world and five million married women are employed in the UK. It's very difficult to find out exactly how many women with young children work because so many of them do part-time work or work at home and much of this goes unrecorded by government agencies. In the USA in 1969 one in four women with children under three was working and in 1971 in this country one in five women with children under four was working, though only one in twenty-five worked full-time. With the inflation that has occurred over the last five years in the UK it seems very likely that many more women with young children are working today.

We saw in chapter 1 how young Western women are brought up to think of themselves as important economic units and how this mitigates against breast feeding in a general sort of way. To many young women, jobs come first and raising children has to fit in with keeping up the family's standard of living. Having said this, though, such figures as are available show that only a tiny proportion of women are working when their children are of breast feeding age.

Let's make no bones about it – full breast feeding and work don't mix – at least not in this country. The International Labour Organization has laid down rules to help mothers breast feed in certain other countries. It stipulates that nursing mothers should have a break of half an hour twice during the working day. These breaks are recognized in many countries and in some the breaks are shorter and more frequent. Two breaks during the day mean that a mother can feed before work, once during the morning, at lunch time, once during the afternoon and then at home in the evening and at night as much as necessary. In many countries employers must by law provide a room for breast feeding mothers. In France, for instance, establishments employing more than 100 women over the age of fifteen must provide nurseries. In Denmark, if twenty-five or more women are employed, a breast feeding room must be provided.

Breast feeding is almost impossible for working mothers in the UK as so few organizations have nurseries. In parts of Africa babies are either brought to the working mother by relatives so that she can feed or the mothers take their babies to work and actually have them by their sides as they work. Neither of these is likely to happen here!

But although it is difficult to combine breast feeding and working, let's see how it can be done. First, though, we'll discuss why women *want* to combine the two.

Many mothers today say that living is so expensive that they simply can't afford to run a home on one income. That may seem to be the case but it's a thought that's worth challenging. Just think what you'd have to go without if you didn't work for nine months, for instance, and weigh up the advantages of being with your baby and feeding him the best way you possibly could. Very often going back to work is shrouded in economic excuses when really the mother wants to keep in the swim, maintain her career or even simply her own self-image. Mothers who take to mothering naturally don't want to leave their babies – they'll go through all sorts of hardships to stay at home. Even taking a part-time job to 'be released from the baby' or to 'keep up one's sanity' and all the other sorry reasons mothers give is a sad but understandable reflection on today's society. With today's small family units and the inevitable isolation of mothers and babies at home, it's not really surprising that many mothers don't enjoy the experience of looking after their children and so try to find a way out.

In rural Africa a mother and her baby are not parted at all for the first fifteen months of life. A sample of these mothers has been studied carefully to see if they get irritated by being with their children so closely for so long. No ill effects could be found in either the mothers or their babies. A popular myth is that babies need exposure to lots of different people to make them sociable. There's no evidence that this is so. Babies need their mothers and they need them most in the first years of life.

Of course there is a small number of women for whom working is essential for the financial survival of the family and many more for whom the extra money would be helpful, so let's be practical and see how breast feeding can be managed while working.

Obviously the easiest solution is to work at home doing something that makes money. There are all kinds of home-based jobs, from making things to telephone selling, which will enable you to carry on feeding naturally. The next best option is to work part-time and locally. If you work part-time and you're producing enough milk you may like to express some to leave in a bottle in the fridge for your baby minder to give your baby while you are out. This can be done in the morning, when many mothers find they have lots of milk, or even the night before, especially if your baby skips a feed at night. Some mothers find they can express enough milk while they're at work to make it worth while storing (preferably in a fridge) to take home and give the baby minder for the next day. The trouble with expressing is that it's rather tedious, usually takes longer than actually feeding the baby and needs privacy and somewhere comfortable to sit. When done in the morning it tends to be rushed because there's so much else to do, so there either may not be enough milk or else you give up after a few days. If you are dedicated enough to carry on you'll have the satisfaction of knowing that your baby is fully breast fed.

With part-time work your baby will possibly only need feeding once while you're away if you work near home. When you work some way away from home or when you're back full-time it's very difficult to leave enough expressed milk for the baby while you're away. This means that he may have to have some cows' milk, which is not ideal in the first four to six months as we've explained.

Being back at work doesn't mean you can't breast feed at all, though. You can still feed before you go and as soon as you come back, besides at night. It's really tiring if you're getting up at night *and* working full-time, so bear this in mind when deciding to go back to work. Once you stop feeding on demand your milk will probably slowly dry up, so with this sort of irregular feeding you'll gradually start weaning your baby whether you like it or not.

Very few women give up breast feeding to go back to work. In a study in Blackburn, only 0.6 per cent of women stopped for this reason. Those who really want to breast feed carry on as long as they want and go back to work later at a time to suit themselves.

So, in summary, if you want to or have to work, do everything you possibly can to stay at home with your baby for at least four to six months, working at home if you can. After four to six months combine breast and bottle feeding if you have to but carry on breast feeding as long as you can, even if it's only one feed a day.

12 Some common problems

Engorgement of the breasts

When your milk starts to come in in the first few days it's very important that your breasts are emptied frequently by the baby in order to prevent them becoming overfilled.

If they are not properly emptied, milk will build up in the ducts until the breasts become swollen, lumpy, hard, tense, painful and hot. This is called engorgement and is due not only to the excess milk but also to the swelling caused by leakage of fluid from lymphatic and blood vessels which have been blocked by the increased pressure in the breasts. This fluid collects under the skin and in the connective tissues. The skin of engorged breasts is liable to bruise and is shiny and pitted like orange peel.

Added to this, the breasts are lumpy and the swollen ducts and milk reservoirs can often be seen standing out beneath the skin.

A mother with engorgement feels hot and shivery and may sweat profusely. She often feels thirsty and should drink according to her thirst, and not limit drinks as she may be advised to do. Some mothers also feel rather weepy when they have engorged breasts. This may be because of the discomfort or may be because engorgement often coincides with the low period often noticed at the end of the first week. Some experts go so far as to say if mothers didn't get engorged breasts, they wouldn't become depressed post-natally.

But discomfort is only a part of the problem. The milk-producing cells within the milk glands are also affected by the high pressure in the breasts. They become flattened and unable to produce so much milk. While this may be a good thing in the short term, in that it reduces milk production and so reduces further build-up of pressure in the breasts, it's a very bad thing in the long term, because the ability of the cells to produce milk can be damaged so much that milk production is shut down altogether.

This is the method most hospitals use to dry up milk in mothers who don't want to feed their babies. They are advised not to feed and their milk simply goes. They become engorged towards the end of the first week, as their milk comes in even without their babies feeding at the breast, but because of the build-up of pressure in their breasts, the milk-producing cells are so damaged that they stop producing milk at all. With no further stimulus from suckling and thus no hormone release, the milk dries up.

The breast feeding mother with a good let-down reflex is lucky as, if she does become engorged, by breast feeding properly she can restore the milk-producing cells to their former, healthy state, so that when she has managed to get rid of the engorgement, her milk production will be as good as before. If she were to carry on breast feeding half-heartedly, the engorgement might be relieved but her milk production might never again regain its former potential, and would eventually dry up.

Poor management of engorgement is one of the commonest reasons for 'failure' of the milk supply in the early days yet this failure should be entirely preventable. Mothers who say that their milk vanished after a week could in almost every case have breast fed successfully if only they had been given better advice.

If you follow the advice earlier in the book about how to manage breast feeding in the first few days, *it's unlikely that you will become engorged at all.* However, if you have been given poor advice (and one leading American doctor says that in his opinion engorgement is a disorder caused by doctors!), then this is how to cope with the engorgement and lay the foundations for successful breast feeding in the months ahead:

1 Feed your baby more often and feed him as soon as your breasts feel at all full, even if he hasn't asked for a feed and is asleep.

2 Feed your baby for longer periods. A good guide is fifteen minutes each side, though we don't like giving lengths of time. If the baby will feed for longer, so much the better.

3 If your breasts are so tense that it's difficult for your baby to feed, soften the areola beforehand by removing some milk. You can do this in one of several ways: by gently expressing a little milk by hand (if this is not too painful); by having a hot bath to encourage leaking; by splashing your breasts with warm water over a hand basin; and by encouraging your let-down to work by relaxing, going through the routine of preparing to feed and by taking an aspirin or a small alcoholic drink to reduce any pain which may be stopping you from letting down your milk.
A baby that is allowed to suck on a tense areola will be unlikely to get the breast into his mouth properly, will chew on a small part of the nipple and not only make the nipple sore but also get very little milk. This is because he is not able to drain the milk reservoirs and the pain he is causing by chewing on the nipples prevents the let-down from working.

4 If your baby is too apathetic (see page 152) to empty the breasts adequately, when he has finished feeding, you can empty them either by hand or with an Egnell breast pump. This electric pump is owned by many hospitals and is more efficient at removing milk than hand pumps. If your hospital doesn't have one, you can hire one from the National Childbirth Trust hiring agents throughout the country (see page 6). They can be bought from Eschmann Brothers & Walsh Ltd, (Matburn Surgical Equipment Division), Peter Road, Lancing, Sussex, but are expensive to buy (over £400)!

5 The tenderness and pain of engorged breasts can be relieved with ice packs or with hot or cold compresses (made by wringing out a face flannel in hot or cold water) applied as often as necessary.

Sore and painful nipples

Many breast feeding mothers experience pain in their nipples during the early weeks of breast feeding, particularly in the first week, and unfortunately this pain puts many of them off completely. Various surveys have estimated that between 13 per cent and 80 per cent of mothers have sore nipples at some time.

Although it's not always possible to prevent the nipples

becoming painful, it is possible to prevent the condition from lasting too long or from getting worse.

What causes the pain? There is some dispute about this, especially as in some women the nipple skin itself is undamaged. In others, the nipple skin is visibly damaged, usually with reddening and raising of the small projections (papillae) of the nipples together with a crescentic stripe of 'petechiae' – tiny spots of blood within the skin – across each nipple. Crusting of the skin can also occur.

The pain from a sore nipple begins as soon as the baby starts feeding and lasts only a minute or two, not throughout the feed. In mothers feeding their babies on demand, the peak of nipple soreness occurs on the third day and by the fourth day it is decreasing, whereas in mothers feeding their babies on a four-hourly schedule, the soreness continues to get worse until the fourth day. Babies fed on a schedule may damage the nipple skin more as they suck more strongly because they are so hungry. Large babies tend to cause more soreness than small ones, for the same reason.

The pain is very characteristic and is described as being as though the baby were biting the nipple. It usually goes as soon as the milk is let down and it is perhaps for this reason that it is always less or even non-existent in the 'second' breast.

The most reasonable explanation for the pain, with or without actual skin damage, would seem to be the suction exerted on the nipple by the baby's mouth before the milk is let down. Very high negative pressures are reached in his mouth during this time, and these are the cause of the skin damage described above. The crescentic stripe actually represents the area of the nipple exposed to maximum suction, the baby's palate resting above the stripe and his tongue below. Mothers who have no visible skin damage may have tougher nipple skin which is more resistant to the suction exerted. The pain stops when the let-down reflex operates because the supply of milk means the baby no longer needs to suck so strongly.

When the milk is being produced freely, towards the end of the first week after birth, there is always some foremilk available for the baby when he is put to the breast and extreme pressure causing damage to the skin from sucking an empty milk reservoir should not occur.

In the occasional mother who experiences soreness of the nipples in later weeks, it is possible that the foremilk is not getting to the baby as soon as he sucks. This may be because her ducts are kept closed because she is cold, in which case she should either have a warm shower or bath before feeding or bathe her breasts with warm water. She should also feed in a warm room.

A baby who has the nipple and areola positioned poorly in his mouth, because of being held awkwardly, poorly protractile nipples or engorgement of the breast, will be more likely to cause soreness due to skin damage.

What can be done to treat sore nipples?

The cardinal rule is to carry on feeding – DON'T STOP, whatever you're told.

1 *First of all and very important make sure that your baby is positioned well at the breast.* If your nipple skin looks sore, with a stripe across it, it's highly likely that he is feeding with his mouth in an awkward position, so exerting unnecessary suction on the nipple to hold it in place. Sit up or even lean slightly forward making sure that the baby is not tugging at the nipple but is well supported. Put the baby's chest against yours, so he doesn't have to turn his head to get to the breast, and make sure his chin is against your breast. He should have part or all of the areola (depending on its size) in his mouth, and certainly not just the nipple itself. Change the position in which you feed your baby during the day, for instance give him some feeds lying down and some with him held under your arm with his feet pointing backwards. This will help ensure that no single part of the nipple takes the force of his suction every time.

2 *If your nipples are poorly protractile,* try using breast shells for half an hour or so before a feed. These may make the nipples temporarily stand out enough for the baby to take them properly. Be careful to keep the shells clean to avoid introducing infection into the damaged skin. A word of warning here, though. Breast shells can make the nipple skin swollen and moist because of the

still, warm, moist air inside them. This may itself cause more soreness and can also make a crack of the nipple skin worse. Whether or not the shells help is an individual matter and the thing is to try them once or twice to see if they help you.

3 *If you are engorged*, treat this as described on page 141. A baby will find it difficult to feed in the correct position from an engorged breast and is very likely to chew the nipple as the areola may be too tense to be taken into his mouth.

4 Fear of pain, as well as actual pain, both delay the let-down reflex, which means that the baby will carry on sucking and your nipples will be painful for longer. Try and *encourage your let-down* to work before the baby is put to the breast by going through a set routine of preparing for a feed.

5 *Feed your baby on demand.* This will encourage the milk to come in sooner and will also aid the establishment of your let-down reflex. You may develop sore nipples sooner than your schedule-feeding neighbour in the next bed but the soreness will also disappear before hers, your breast feeding will almost certainly be more successful and you will be less likely to develop mastitis.

6 *Don't limit drinking time but limit total suckling time.* Suckling to comfort your baby while he goes to sleep after he's finished drinking is good practice when your nipples are *not* sore but you may find it helps healing if you take him off the breast at this stage in the first week or so if you have sore nipples. By doing this and by encouraging your let-down to work before he feeds (number 4 above) you'll limit total suckling time but not actual drinking time.

7 *Care for your nipple skin* as described on page 97 and be careful not to soak your nipples in the bath water for too long. Moisture makes soreness last longer, especially if the baby feeds on soggy nipple skin, as the skin is more liable to damage after being soaked.

8 Some authorities recommend using an *antiseptic cream* (Cetavlex cream) on sore nipple skin to help prevent a fissure developing. Rotersept spray may also be useful.

9 Always *offer the less sore nipple first*. By the time you offer the sore one, your milk should be flowing well and there should be little pain.

10 *Take an aspirin or a small alcholic drink* a short time before a feed if you feel the pain is inhibiting your let-down.

11 Careful use of a *sun lamp* can speed up the healing of damaged nipple skin. You should be four feet away from the lamp and your eyes protected by goggles. Expose your nipples for half a minute on the first day, one minute on days two and three, two minutes on days four and five and three minutes on day six. If there is any reddening of the skin, reduce the exposure time. If you can sunbathe with your nipples exposed, the sunlight will help a lot. If you have no garden, sunbathe indoors with the window open. Failing a sun lamp or sunlight, try exposing your nipples to the light from an electric light bulb.

12 *Don't remove any crusts* appearing on the nipples – they are part of the healing process.

13 Some people advocate using a *nipple shield* over the sore nipple. This has a teat for the baby to suck the milk through. It may or may not help – try it if all the other measures fail. One danger is that if not properly cleaned between times it can introduce infection into the damaged skin and cause a fissure. Rubber 'Natural Nursing Nipple Shields' are available from the National Childbirth Trust Breast Feeding Promotion Group Headquarters. It's important not to use such a shield for long because milk production and the establishment of the let-down depend on actual skin stimulation by the baby.

14 Last, but no means least, is to *expose your nipples to the air* as much as possible. You may think this is difficult in our cold climate and with our culture, but you can sleep naked at night and leave your bra off during the day to allow the air to circulate under your top clothes. Once the soreness has healed, wear your bra again.

Air helps tremendously because it dries the nipple skin. If sore nipple skin is allowed to remain moist after a feed, the soreness will persist. Moisture also makes cracking more likely. When you wear a bra again, dry your nipples before covering them, and if you use anything inside your bra to mop up leaks, make sure it is changed frequently to stop the nipples being enclosed in soggy material for long periods.

Rarely, a sore nipple may bleed and the baby may swallow tiny amounts of blood. This can look horrifying if it's regurgitated in a mouthful of milk. There's no need to worry about this. Your blood is quite harmless to the baby. Treat the soreness and carry on feeding.

If nipple soreness persists for the whole feed, it may be caused by dermatitis from detergents used to wash clothing or from substances in creams or other remedies applied to your nipples. Once the cause has been tracked down, remove it and treat the nipples with hydrocortisone cream from your doctor.

Nipple fissures or cracks

A few women develop a fissure or crack in the nipple usually after the fifth day. This develops at the base of the nipple and may follow poor treatment of the more usual nipple soreness described above. A fissure is acutely painful and needs careful and prompt treatment if the pain is not going to put the woman off breast feeding altogether. Thrush, possibly from the baby's mouth, may infect the fissure and will need special treatment.

The best prevention and treatment for a fissure is to take all the steps for the treatment of sore nipples. If, however, you have a fissure which doesn't heal with this treatment within a few days, you'll probably find it necessary to take the baby off the breast because of the pain and either express the milk or use an Egnell pump for a while – sometimes as long as four or five days, though usually for only one or two. When the fissure has healed, gradually resume feeding your baby, starting twice a day and continuing to pump or express regularly in between feeds. Some mothers find they can continue to feed if they use a nipple shield, but again, great care must be taken to keep it clean and to stop using it as soon as possible.

Blocked duct
This causes a red, tender lump in the breast. The duct becomes blocked either because of pressure from part of a badly fitting bra or from generalized engorgement of the breasts with inadequate emptying of one duct in particular. Milk builds up in the duct behind the blockage and causes a lump. When the baby feeds, the let-down works even in the area of the breast supplying the blocked duct, so the pressure builds up more, making the lump often at its most painful as the milk lets down.

Milk escapes from the duct into the surrounding tissues of the breast and causes reddening of the overlying skin. Some also gets into the bloodstream and makes the body temperature rise. This can cause a fever as high as 104°F after a feed. The mother may feel 'flu-like and achy as well.

Treatment of a blocked duct should be regarded as urgent because stagnant milk can so easily become infected, causing mastitis. Simple measures, started at the first suspicion that anything is wrong, should do the trick in every case.

1 Make sure the whole breast is emptied thoroughly each time the baby feeds. Let him feed as long as he wants and then express any residual milk.

2 Should your breasts or even a part of a breast still feel lumpy after a feed, feed the baby more often to ensure frequent drainage of the ducts. Try and fit in as many extra feeds as you can, even if you are already feeding on demand.

3 Offer the affected breast first to ensure best possible emptying.

4 *Gently* massage the lump towards the nipple after a feed if it is still there, in an attempt to empty it.

5 Check that your bra is not pressing anywhere and so causing the block, especially if you're using one of the nursing bras that has a band across the top of the breast when the flap is open.

6 Vary the position of your baby at each feed.

7 Relieve the pain with hot or cold compresses applied every hour or put a hot water bottle over the area.

8 Take aspirin to relieve the pain if necessary.

9 If the lump is still present after twenty-four hours in spite of all these measures, it's wise to take a course of antibiotics to prevent the onset of mastitis, so go and see your doctor. *You don't have to stop feeding.*

10 Make sure you get plenty of rest. Actually go to bed; even if it's only for one day it will make you feel better and may help keep your resistance up so that your blocked duct won't lead to mastitis.

Mastitis

Poor or delayed treatment of a blocked duct can lead to mastitis – infection of the breast. The infection develops in the milk which has escaped from the duct into the breast tissue, so the infection isn't present in the duct itself.

The appearance of an infected breast differs only in degree from that of the breast with a blocked duct. The infected area is red, swollen, hot and painful, with shiny skin, and the mother feels shivery and 'flu-like as before.

The treatment of mastitis is as for a blocked duct, with the addition of an antibiotic. There is *no* danger to the baby from drinking the milk, as the organisms responsible are not harmful and in any case are rarely present in the milk.

Don't be tempted or persuaded to wean your baby – if you do you'll be likely to develop a breast abscess.

This sort of mastitis, known as *sporadic mastitis*, is most often seen after several weeks of breast feeding. Occasionally it occurs without a duct being blocked, apparently out of the blue.

Epidemic mastitis

This is another type of infection which is passed to the breast from the baby and causes illness in the first two weeks or so of feeding. The organisms responsible often come from the hospital nursery and are carried in the baby's nose. Several mothers and babies may be affected at once in a hospital, hence the name 'epidemic' mastitis.

The infection involves the milk ducts (not the tissues outside the ducts as with mastitis following a blocked duct), and it is often possible to squeeze pus from the nipple. The breast is red, hot, tender and swollen and the mother feels feverish and ill.

The organisms responsible are from a more virulent strain of *Staphylococcus aureus* than that causing sporadic mastitis and may be sensitive to one of the newer penicillins though some are penicillin-resistant. A milk sample should be cultured by the laboratory to determine which antibiotic is most suitable. The baby will probably come to no harm from drinking the infected milk if you are taking antibiotics though some researchers suggest that milk with large numbers of dead or alive bacteria may produce a toxic or irritant effect (such as gastro-enteritis or even septicaemia) in the baby and that the milk should not be drunk, even after sterilizing. A mother's milk, even if infected with these organisms, is probably tolerated better by her own baby than by someone else's. To be absolutely safe in cases of epidemic mastitis, a sample of milk should be examined and if found to contain a high bacteria count the baby should only be fed from the other breast or should have milk from another mother, or cows' milk if no breast milk is available. The breast should be emptied well and often, by expression or pumping, to maintain the milk supply and you should rest as much as possible. Treat the pain with aspirin, hot or cold compresses and relax as much as you can before a feed to aid your let-down. If the bacteria count of the milk is within safe limits, or when it drops to safe limits, nursing can be continued, but until then the milk should be discarded.

Breast abscess

This is usually preventable as it follows mastitis which has been poorly treated. One survey showed that *abscesses only occurred in women who stopped feeding when they got mastitis.* The lump is not tender.

Treatment is as for epidemic mastitis but if the abscess doesn't resolve, surgical drainage will be necessary. Needless to say you shouldn't feed the baby from the affected breast – simply carry on with the other breast and temporarily discard the expressed milk from the one with the abscess.

After this catalogue of horrors the reader could be forgiven for thinking that she's going to have all kinds of unpleasant problems with swollen breasts and abscesses. This of course is not the case.

The complications we've mentioned here are uncommon (except for sore nipples) and almost unknown in women who breast feed solely on demand right from the beginning. A doctor we know who worked in a totally breast feeding hospital unit in Africa saw no mastitis or breast abscesses in four years of looking after several thousand mothers.

Contrast this with the Western world where an average of 9 per cent of breast feeding mothers get mastitis, 5 to 11 per cent of whom suffer from breast abscesses.

Difficult feeders

Some babies take to the breast within a few minutes of being born and never give their mothers any trouble. Others, however, seem completely uninterested, feed briefly then let go and cry, or even seem to have a battle with the breast. In nearly every case there is a reason for the baby's behaviour. Let's look at the possible causes in turn.

Babies affected by mother's pain-killers in labour. In this country pethidine is a common offender, while in the USA many babies are affected by barbiturates given to the mother in labour. These babies may be drowsy and apathetic about feeding for up to five days, though the effects usually wear off more quickly. Good obstetric care includes not giving large doses of analgesics shortly before the birth.

You might not be able to get your sedated baby to feed well but you can stop him being given a bottle and you can keep your milk supply going by expressing or pumping milk after each feed. You can also try giving him expressed milk from a spoon when he has finished feeding. Wake him often – every two or three hours at least – for a feed, as the sooner he learns how to feed from your breast, the better. While you or a nurse may be able to get him to suck from a bottle even if he won't feed from you, this isn't a good idea as he'll be far less likely to take to the breast once the sedation has worn off.

The keynote to coping with this problem is perseverance but you can cope if you know what to do.

Poor feeding position. If the baby is not correctly positioned at the breast, the nipple will not be taken far enough into the mouth and the stimulus to feed will not be strong enough. See page 93 to make sure you are giving him the best chance to feed properly.

Inadequate nipples. A few mothers still have poorly protractile nipples at the end of their pregnancies, though these tend to improve once the baby has been suckled for several weeks. You'll find it helps to wear breast shells for half an hour or so before a feed – this brings the nipples out just long enough for the baby to get a hold. A similar effect can be produced by a breast pump. Once he has 'latched on', the nipple should stay out for the length of the feed. When he stops feeding, though, it'll go back in.

You can also help your baby to latch on by taking your nipple and areola between your finger and thumb and making a 'biscuit' for him to take hold of.

A rubber nipple shield can help in some cases in the early days but should be discarded as soon as possible as the nipples need the stimulus of suckling.

Engorgement (see page 142)

Tired baby. If you are made to feed your baby according to a schedule in hospital, he may cry from hunger for some time – perhaps as long as an hour – before you are given him to feed. This is especially likely to happen at visiting times and at night. By the time you get him he is exhausted and goes to sleep after feeding for a very short time, even sometimes before your milk lets down.

Obviously this situation is ridiculous. You must insist, or get your husband to insist, that you are given your baby as soon as he cries. Remember that the smaller the baby, the more often he'll need feeding and the sooner crying will exhaust him.

Full baby. If your baby is given a cows' milk complement after you have fed him, he's unlikely to be hungry by the time the hospital decrees he's ready for a feed from you. This is because cows' milk stays in the stomach for much longer than breast milk. You'll know by this stage that complements are rarely, if ever, necessary in the first weeks, so tell the sister that you would rather feed your baby more often and for longer and that you don't want him to have anything other than breast milk to drink, day or night. Remember that you need your baby to feed often so that your milk comes in quickly. A satisfied baby is no help to your breasts as he simply won't feed.

Baby kept from you after birth. The best time to start suckling is in the first half an hour after birth. After this the baby's urge to feed gradually lessens, though of course you can still teach your baby with patience. Learning to feed is best done in the first few hours – after that you'll have a much slower pupil on your hands.

Jaundiced baby. A jaundiced baby is often sleepy and difficult to interest in feeding. Frequent small feeds are the best for him. As the jaundice clears, his interest will increase, so be patient and maintain your milk supply by expressing after each feed if necessary.

Baby has been given a bottle. A baby who has sucked from a rubber teat will find it more difficult to feed from you as the teat is such a 'supernormal' stimulus. You can get him to feed from you with patience but keep him away from that bottle! Once a baby has fed from the breast for many weeks, the occasional experience of sucking from a teat shouldn't matter, though some babies very quickly learn that milk comes from a bottle more easily and are reluctant to take the breast if there's the slightest chance of getting a bottle.

Baby fights at the breast. A baby who fights at the breast has probably had one experience of being smothered by the full breast while feeding and has learnt that, for him, getting milk means not getting air through his nose. Make sure that your breast is not obstructing his nose. You may have to hold your breast away with your opposite hand. With patience on your part he'll forget his early unpleasant experience.

Don't confuse fighting at the breast with the very common playing and butting some babies do while they're waiting for the milk to let down. These babies are perfectly happy once the milk is flowing, whereas the true fighters carry on fighting and never seem to feed properly.

If your baby is still reluctant to take the breast, try the trick of popping a rubber teat – perhaps filled with expressed milk – into his mouth. Once he latches on, withdraw it and substitute your nipple.

Whatever the cause of the difficulty with feeding, make sure that you keep your milk supply going. Though a few babies never feed enthusiastically, they all feed eventually if given the chance. The feeding of an unenthusiastic baby may not be enough to stimulate your milk supply, so it's up to you to express or pump after each feed. You may need to keep this up for some weeks, so be prepared.

Baby refuses one breast. Occasionally a baby will seem to take a liking to one breast and refuse to feed from the other. This may be because he is more comfortable on one side or because the milk seems to come more easily from that breast. To overcome this, try feeding him from the side he likes best first, so that the milk is flowing from the other side, then transfer him to the other breast without turning him round, so letting him feed in the 'twin' position. This may do the trick. If not, express milk from the unused breast to maintain its milk supply and keep trying at each feed time. He'll almost certainly come round to the idea of feeding from both sides again.

Baby overwhelmed by milk supply. If your let-down is so strong that the milk gushes into your baby's mouth and nearly chokes him, you will find it helps if you collect this early milk in a sterilized container and only allow your baby to continue feeding when the milk has stopped flowing so exuberantly. If necessary you can give him the collected milk by spoon afterwards.

Babies who manage to swallow quickly enough to cope with such an exuberant milk supply may swallow too much air with the milk and so develop colic or regurgitate more than usual after a feed. Some babies in fact bring up almost a whole feed like this. Expressing or just collecting the initial milk you let down as described above should get over this problem. If you simply allow the baby to bring up a whole feed and then feed him again, he'll certainly keep the milk down because the flow will be much slower and he won't swallow so much air, but your milk supply will increase because of the law of supply and demand, and your let-down will work even better, so making the problem worse at the next feed. One way of overcoming the problem of too much milk is to give one breast per feed, letting the baby suck on the empty breast for comfort. (See page 109.) Give the other breast at the next feed. This allows the baby to suck for comfort without getting two breasts full of milk at each feed. Express some milk from the unused breast to keep you comfortable if necessary.

Premature babies

One of the most difficult feeding situations is when you have a very small baby which has been born early (pre-term). Generally, the more immature the baby, the less powerful is the urge to feed and the more perseverance is needed on your part to keep up your milk supply until the baby grows large enough to suck more strongly.

Technically, a premature baby is one weighing less than five and a half pounds (2,500 g), though even five- and six-pound babies may not feed as well as bigger ones. A pre-term baby weighing less than two or three pounds will not have a sucking reflex at all and will have to be tube fed. As he matures, the sucking reflex will gradually appear and you can begin to suckle him. Occasionally, a baby may be small and yet full term (small-for-dates) – he may have been poorly nourished in the uterus. In this case he may have a sucking reflex in spite of weighing very little so it's worth asking the doctors looking after your baby whether you should try suckling, whatever the weight of the baby, unless you know that the baby was born weeks before the expected date.

Premature babies do best on breast milk and indeed many hospitals give them breast milk from a milk bank if their mothers don't want to give them their own milk. The breast milk is given by a fine tube passed down the nose and back of the throat into the gullet and thence the stomach. This tube stays where it is between feeds. Breast milk given in this way is usually best pumped from the mother's breasts with an Egnell electric pump, though it can be manually expressed if a pump is temporarily unavailable. Hand expression takes longer and is not always as effective in producing large volumes of milk as a pump is. Although your tiny baby won't need large volumes for some time, you need to empty your breasts as fully as possible at short, regular intervals in order to keep up a good milk supply. It's just as important to collect your milk soon after birth as it would be if you had a baby of normal size, and just as important to prevent problems such as engorgement.

Premature babies are nursed in incubators in special care nurseries to keep them warm and protect them from infection. This means that you will have to go to your baby when you want to see him, though someone else can collect your milk and take it to him. Physical contact is very important for the development of the mothering instinct, which isn't always spontaneous by any means. If the staff will let you, hold your baby as often as you can, or at least stroke him gently through the armholes in the incubator.

As soon as the baby has grown mature enough to breast feed, you can offer him your breast. At first he may not succeed and you'll need to persevere for some days or perhaps even weeks, keeping your milk supply going in the meantime. If you have to return home without your baby, you can hire an Egnell pump to use at home from the National Childbirth Trust and deliver your milk to the hospital each day when you visit.

Breast milk banks

In 1975 there were only five proper milk banks in England and Wales (London, Cardiff, Birmingham, Bristol and Brighton) though more are being set up. Milk is supplied to these banks by nursing mothers with milk to spare and can be transported by road or rail if necessary to premature or sick babies in hospitals with no access to donated breast milk.

Donor mothers are screened carefully before their milk is accepted. Their past medical history, blood tests and drug intake are carefully noted. If the mother is taking any drugs, including nicotine, alcohol, aspirin and the Pill, her milk is not accepted.

The donated milk is refrigerated, then collected daily, cultured to make sure the bacteria count is low enough, pasteurized if necessary and frozen for a maximum of six months. The pasteurization is best done by the 'flash' method to decrease the inactivation of antibodies and enzymes. Ideally, donated breast milk is used without being sterilized at all. Breast milk from these banks has helped save the lives of many sick or tiny babies whose own mothers could not or would not feed them themselves.

If you have milk to spare and are prepared to donate it to other babies, mention this to your health visitor, doctor, breast feeding counsellor or hospital sister. They will probably be delighted.

The baby with teeth

Some babies are actually born with one or two teeth, though most don't get a tooth for the first six months at least. There is no reason why teeth should interfere with breast feeding as the baby's gums are not used for feeding – the pressure comes from the tongue below and the palate above.

Your baby may, however, try the odd bite when he's older and will be very interested in your reaction. It's best to say 'no' firmly and gently take him off the breast. If you smile, he may think you like it and do it again! Some babies only bite towards the end of a feed and this is easily handled. Simply take him off the breast before he starts to bite . . . you'll soon get to know when he's about to do it.

Some mothers have found a rubber nipple shield useful if their baby likes to bite.

Finally, remember that some babies bite from frustration if the breast is too full or if there is not enough milk. You can cope with this sort of biting by dealing with the underlying problem.

13 Some special situations

Baby ill or in hospital

Unless your baby is so ill that he is not allowed any milk, he'll do better with your milk than with any other and will make a faster recovery after such illnesses as gastro-enteritis if his bowel doesn't have to cope with cows' milk.

If he has to go into hospital, the ideal is for you to go too so you can be near him to comfort and support him emotionally and also to feed him. If you can spend the day with him but can't stay at night, then leave as much expressed or pumped milk as you can for the nurses to give him from a spoon (or from a bottle if you are confident that he will not learn to prefer the bottle).

If you can visit only infrequently you may need to bring enough milk for a whole day. This requires patience to do day after day but can be done and is easiest if you can borrow an Egnell breast pump to use at home.

Most hospitals allow unrestricted visiting of children but if your hospital tries to stop you coming in when you like, explain that you're breast feeding and that it's very important for your baby and for your milk supply that you visit when you like. Most hospitals will cooperate once they understand your feelings.

When your baby has his injections at the doctor's surgery or clinic he may go off his food and be more fussy than usual for about twenty-four hours. If you're getting over full because he's not eating well, simply express a little milk. You'll need to do this whenever he wants less food for a day or two when he's off colour.

If your baby is jaundiced

There are many causes for jaundice (yellow colouring of the skin) in the first few weeks of life, ranging from the harmless 'physiological' jaundice which many babies get, to jaundice from rhesus incompatibility, which can be serious if not treated adequately. The diagnosis depends on the time of onset of the jaundice and on the results of blood tests.

Breast milk jaundice

Very rarely a baby develops jaundice from breast milk. This jaundice disappears within three to seven days if he is weaned on to cows' milk. This sort of jaundice is luckily not harmful to the baby, so there is no reason why breast feeding should be stopped. It is, of course, important for an accurate diagnosis to be made so as to rule out any more serious causes of the jaundice. Breast milk jaundice tends to appear towards the end of the first week of life, becomes worst from the seventh to tenth day and lasts from three weeks to two months.

Rhesus antibodies

Many mothers who know they have rhesus antibodies in their blood worry that if they breast feed, these antibodies may be passed to the baby via the milk. Rhesus antibodies are present in breast milk if present in the mother's blood but they have no effect on the baby because they are inactivated in his gut. It is therefore quite safe to breast feed your rhesus positive baby if you are rhesus negative and have rhesus antibodies, even if he is jaundiced. Indeed, it's the best way to feed these babies, according to several studies.

A jaundiced baby is more drowsy than normal so you may find you have trouble in feeding. Your baby should not be allowed to cry for long periods before a feed as this will tire him still further. Feed him frequently, waking him if necessary for a feed.

If for any reason your milk is slow to come in, your baby may need extra drinks of water to prevent dehydration which could raise the levels of bilirubin in the blood supply to the brain.

The baby with cleft lip and/or palate

The initial shock of discovering that your baby has a cleft lip, with or without a cleft palate, may make you reluctant to breast feed. If you can get over this initial feeling of disappointment, you'll remember that you never see older children walking around with any noticeable deformity of their lips. The plastic surgery available today is so good that the defect can be almost perfectly repaired.

Many units are now repairing these clefts within two days of birth, though others still wait the traditional three months before operating. Early surgery is by far the best from the feeding point of view, as not only does it make feeding easier for the baby but it also makes the mother emotionally more inclined to breast feed, because her baby looks normal. During these first few days, until the lips have healed well enough for your baby to breast feed, keep your milk supply going by frequent expression or pumping, preferably with an electric pump. The milk can be given to the baby in a specially shaped spoon.

If it's decided to postpone the operation for several months, you'll need a lot of patience while feeding, as babies with a cleft lip often find it difficult to suck well and take a long time over their feeds. If the baby has a severe cleft and you find it impossible to breast feed, you can still give him your milk from a specially shaped spoon or a bottle with an adapted teat. Ask your paediatrician about these.

The mentally handicapped baby

There is every reason why you should breast feed your mentally handicapped baby – he will get the same benefits from being breast fed as any other baby and it will help cement the bond between you. Unfortunately some of these babies feed rather apathetically and so take a long time over their feeds but a bottle feed would be just as time-consuming. With patience you'll succeed and you'll be sure you're doing the best for your baby. Many women with handicapped babies feel that they deserve every possible help and chance in life and breast feeding is the best starting point.

Mother ill

If you are ill at home and have to be in bed, you'll need someone to look after you and the baby and bring the baby to you when he is ready for a feed (assuming you are too unwell to have him in bed with you). If you have to go into hospital, you may be able to take the baby with you – but this will depend on what is wrong with you, on the hospital's rules and facilities and whether you can have your own room. If you can't have your baby with you, then it may be possible for someone to bring him to you for feeds, though this entails a lot of work and means that you need to be in a hospital close to your home.

Yet another way of carrying on breast feeding if you're in hospital is to express or pump milk and send it home for the baby. It should be stored in the ward refrigerator until collected by a friend or relative to be given the baby by spoon.

There are few illnesses which actually rule out breast feeding. Others do so because of the drugs used to treat them. If you have a *chronic illness* such as severe asthma or kidney disease, you may feel so permanently tired and run down that you couldn't cope with nursing your baby as well. Some mothers manage though, and find that the feeding times make them rest and so tire them less than bottle feeding would.

Diabetic mothers can breast feed and the feeding should make no difference to their insulin requirements if they eat correspondingly more to make up for the calorie loss in milk. Some doctors find that their patients are more stable when breast feeding than they were before. Doctors who deal a lot with diabetic mothers find that they seem to have more difficulty in producing enough milk than non-diabetic women but this is only a generalization and many diabetic mothers feed perfectly satisfactorily.

If you have had *pulmonary tuberculosis* and have been free from disease for two years, you can feed your baby quite safely. If the disease is still active and you are taking anti-tuberculous drugs, then it's quite possible to breast feed and is still good for the baby. Studies in Africa show that the baby should be protected with anti-tuberculous drugs to prevent infection and should also be given a special type of BCG vaccine. The old-fashioned regime for mothers with active TB was either to separate them from their babies or to insist on bottle feeding – this latter was obviously nonsense as the baby was in just as close contact from the point of view of catching a respiratory disease as was a breast fed baby.

Mothers with severe deficiency of Vitamin B_1 (thiamine) causing the disease *beri-beri* should not breast feed their babies as toxic substances are present in the milk. This condition is thankfully not seen in the Western world, though it still exists in parts of China.

Many babies today are born by *Caesarian section* and often the mother will not have been prepared for this method of delivery. After this operation there is no reason why you shouldn't breast feed but you'll need to be extra determined in the first week or so. There are two main problems. Firstly, you're likely to have a certain amount of abdominal pain and discomfort because a Caesar is a serious abdominal operation. This discomfort may make you feel very unmotherly towards your baby. If you are to get your milk supply going well, though, you must feed your baby frequently, just as you would had you had a normal delivery. It's really just as easy to feed the baby as it is to express or pump your milk and you are less likely to have the added problems of engorgement and sore nipples if you feed on demand from the beginning. You'll also prevent your baby from having cows' milk. Of course, you may not be able to feed your baby immediately after delivery as you may have had a general anaesthetic but as soon as you are fully awake, ask for your baby to be brought to you for a feed, even if he is asleep. More Caesarian sections are being performed today under epidural anaesthesia which means that breast feeding gets off to a better start.

The second problem is also related to your operation. You'll find it uncomfortable to feed in the normal sitting position with the baby on your lap. Enlist the help of a nurse at each feed time to position the baby next to you as you are lying down on one side in bed. When the time comes to change breasts, you may be able to leave him on that side and just lean towards him more to offer the other breast. This may not be comfortable though, so ring for a nurse to help you turn over and bring the baby to your other side.

By the end of the first week you should be feeling very much better and will be able to carry on just like any other breast feeding mother.

If your Caesarian baby is nursed in an incubator after delivery and isn't allowed to come to you for feeds, you should express or pump colostrum and milk when it comes in. The nurses will give the breast milk feeds by tube or spoon, depending on the state of the baby. Don't be alarmed by the small amounts of colostrum – remember there isn't much in the first day or so. Remember the special importance of colostrum to your baby.

Drug treatment

Virtually every drug a mother takes will pass into her breast milk, though some reach much higher concentrations than others. Many drugs are harmless to the breast fed baby however high the concentration in the milk, while others may be potentially harmful even in tiny amounts, either because of known side-effects which affect adults as well, or because they have a different action in a small baby than in an older person.

Some drugs can cause the development of sensitivity or allergy which may be dangerous when repeated doses are taken.

Our knowledge of the effects of many drugs on the breast fed baby is far from complete because of the difficulty in doing drug trials in breast feeding mothers. These are difficult because so few breast feeding mothers are actually taking any one drug and it would be wrong to experiment by giving them potentially harmful drugs. There is also the very real difficulty of measuring the levels of drugs in milk and finally there's a general lack of interest in the whole subject, especially since the numbers of breast feeding mothers have fallen over the very years that drug treatment has increased.

Ideally, a breast feeding mother should not take any drugs while she is nursing. However, this is obviously the counsel of perfection and there may be times when drugs will be life-saving and she'll have to take them. If they happen to be dangerous for the baby, then she'll have to wean. There are other drugs which are not life-saving to the mother but are very useful in treating some illnesses. If the particular drug suggested is not safe for the breast fed baby, there is often an alternative which is. Occasionally, the known risks are so low that the mother and her doctor will feel justified in her carrying on with breast feeding while she's taking the drug.

Rather than list the many drugs known to be safe to the breast fed infant, we'll mention the ones that are known to be *either unsafe or better avoided*. If you have any doubts at all – ask your doctor; he can contact the manufacturer of the drug for more details.

Cytotoxic drugs (anti-cancer drugs). You should not breast feed.

Antithyroid drugs. These may cause goitre in the baby which can be treated by giving him thyroxine. However, some also have the relatively rare side-effect of causing a potentially fatal blood disorder. You and your doctor will need to weigh up the risks carefully before you breast feed. Iodides (found in some cough medicines) may also suppress the baby's thyroid activity.

Radio-active isotopes. You should not breast feed. An exception can be made if you have to have a radio-active iodine test: stop breast feeding for seventy-two hours afterwards and discard the breast milk produced during this time. You should have no contact with the baby for six hours after the test. During the seventy-two hours your baby will either have to have donated milk from a friendly nursing mother or from a milk bank, or you will have to give cows' milk.

Steroids. Insufficient studies have been done in humans but animal work shows that it is dangerous for baby rats to receive milk from mother rats on steroids – the sucklings suffer from growth retardation and may die. So it seems safest not to breast feed.

Anticoagulants (blood-thinning drugs). Because of one or two cases of near-death in babies breast fed by mothers taking oral anticoagulants, it used to be advisable not to breast feed. It's now known however that oral warfarin is quite safe, as is heparin by injection.

Chloramphenicol (an anti-infective drug) should be avoided.

Carbamazepine should be avoided.

Nalidixic acid (an anti-infective drug) should be avoided by a breast feeding mother while her baby is very young.

Sulphonamides, cotrimoxazole and all the tetracyclines (anti-infective drugs) should be avoided by the breast feeding mother as they can cause jaundice in the baby. Tetracyclines can cause staining of the teeth in the baby and sulphonamides can cause rashes. Other antibiotics such as penicillin can cause sensitivity reactions in some babies.

Bromides should be avoided by a breast feeding mother as they can cause rashes and drowsiness in the baby.

Ergot-containing medicines (some migraine treatments) should be avoided. The single dose of ergometrine given to a mother to contract her uterus after delivery is safe.

Novobiocin (an antibiotic) should be avoided.

Lead in the form of skin ointments should be avoided.

Mercury. If there is any suspicion that a breast feeding mother has taken this (as happened in Japan when contaminated fish caused the Minamata disease) she should not breast feed.

Oral contraceptives should be avoided. They reduce the milk supply and may have far-reaching but as yet unknown effects on the baby. The progestogen-only Pill is thought not to reduce the milk supply but it may have unknown long-term effects on the baby. (See page 123 for details of contraception.)

Atropine reduces milk production and so should be avoided.

Aspirin in large doses can cause rashes and gastro-intestinal side-effects in the baby. If this happens, you should stop breast feeding. In some cases there is an alternative drug which can be used.

Nicotine (in cigarettes) should be avoided by the breast feeding mother as it may reduce her milk supply.

Dihydrotachysterol. You should not breast feed.

It is safe to drink small amounts of alcohol while breast feeding and *caffeine* (in coffee and tea) is also safe. Amounts of alcohol large enough to make you 'tipsy' have been shown to reduce oxytocin levels and so hinder breast feeding. *Chocolate* may cause rashes in a breast fed baby.

The only laxatives known to have any laxative effect in the breast fed baby are those containing *1, 8-dihydroxyanthraquinone*. *Senna*, *cascara* and the *stool softeners* are without effect on the baby.

A mother breast feeding a baby who may be at risk from developing asthma, eczema or hay fever (that is a baby born into a family with a history of these disorders) should be careful not to overindulge in any food which might be a potential allergen. Many protein foods get into breast milk in amounts which, though small, are nevertheless capable of sensitizing the baby. Foods to avoid *in excess* are eggs, milk, cereal, nuts and fish.

Radio-active fallout. There have been no proven cases of toxicity to breast fed babies from strontium 89 or 90 and caesium 137. Breast milk, in any case, has lower levels of these substances than cows' milk.

DDT presents no problem to the breast fed baby (although it is present in breast milk) because the amounts involved are so small.

If you are taking any drug while you're breast feeding, check with your doctor that it is not one of the above list. Of course, it's wisest always to remind your doctor that you are breast feeding before he prescribes anything for you, as he may not know. Apart from the above list, the vast majority of drugs are thought to be quite safe to take while you're feeding.

Twins

Because two babies demand twice as much milk as one, you'll automatically make enough milk for them. Many mothers have breast fed twins successfully and happily for as long as they wanted to, so don't let anyone try to persuade you that you'll have to give either one or both of them cows' milk.

To save time it's a good idea to get the knack of feeding them both at once, though there will be times when you'll enjoy the luxury of feeding them separately. To feed them together, hold each one with his legs under your arm – cushions or pillows under their heads will take the weight off your arms. Make sure that you position them properly as your nipples may become sore if either baby is dragging on the breast. Once you get into the swing of feeding them both, you'll find it works well.

Should you alternate the breast that each twin feeds from? The usual advice is yes, so that the twin that sucks more strongly has the chance to stimulate each breast alternatively. However, baby animals usually choose 'their' nipple and stick to it, so it may be that human babies would prefer to do just that too. Certainly in the first few weeks of breast feeding, if you always fed one baby from one breast and the other from the other, and if one baby sucked more strongly and so drank more milk each time, then you would find that your breasts were rather lopsided. Once the milk supply is established, the breasts almost always become more equal in size, so this difference is scarcely noticeable.

Should you wake the second baby for a feed every time the first baby wakes? The answer is yes, if you want to save time on feeds and no, if you would like the occasional chance to suckle one baby at a time. If you are at all unhappy about your milk supply then you should always wake the second baby and feed them both.

Re-starting your milk supply

There are two reasons why you might want to do this. Firstly, you may have decided initially not to breast feed, only to change your mind after a few weeks. Secondly, you may want to breast feed an adopted baby. In both cases it's possible to build up your milk supply, though you'll need to persevere and also you'll need a cooperative baby!

If your baby has been on cows' milk for several weeks and your milk supply has dried up, the way to start it up again is by putting the baby to your breast frequently during the day. He may become very frustrated at feeding from an empty breast, especially because the shape of the nipple is not such a strong stimulus to suck as the shape of a rubber teat. You can try two things. Either let him have some cows' milk from the bottle to allay his initial hunger pangs, then let him feed from you, or give him cows' milk from a spoon, so avoiding the stimulus of the teat, then let him feed from you.

After each feed, express or pump your breasts to encourage the milk supply to build up. Remember that the more often the baby breast feeds, the more quickly your milk will re-appear. After about two weeks you will probably produce enough milk for him, so you can do away with cows' milk.

The keynote to success is confidence. Your breasts are quite capable of producing milk again even after several years of being dry, *as long as they have enough stimulation.*

A more unusual situation is if you want to breast feed an adopted baby. Believe it or not, many women have fully breast fed adopted babies years after feeding their own babies, and some women have fed adopted babies without ever having been pregnant, though they needed to supplement the breast milk with other food.

Once your breasts have been prepared for lactation by a pregnancy they will always retain their ability to produce milk. If they have produced milk for any length of time, they'll be even more able to produce milk years later. This is how grandmothers in many parts of the world have breast fed their grandchildren years after feeding their own children.

If you want to build up your milk supply several years after being pregnant or having breast fed your own child, start before the adopted baby arrives, expressing or pumping your breasts at frequent intervals. When the baby arrives, you'll probably need to give both cows' milk and your own milk unless he is lucky enough to have been breast fed until then by his mother. In this case you may be able to carry on giving him breast milk either from her, from a breast milk bank or a friendly breast feeding neighbour, until your milk becomes plentiful enough.

A useful piece of equipment for re-lactating mothers is the Lact-aid, which was developed by a man for his wife who successfully built up her milk supply to feed an adopted baby. This gadget delivers milk from a plastic bag (which you secure to your clothing above your breast) through a fine plastic tube which enters the baby's mouth with your nipple. It can be hired from La Leche League. Because the baby receives milk from the tube while feeding at your breast, he is happy and so continues feeding without getting frustrated. Your nipples also get the necessary stimulation to build up your milk supply.

How long will it take to build up your milk supply? It has been done within two weeks by mothers who weaned their own baby as long as six years before. It usually takes much longer. The pleasure it can give far outweighs the difficulty involved, though you must be prepared for it to take some time.

14 Mainly for fathers

It's probably fair to say that the average husband doesn't care much whether his wife breast feeds or not. This is a pity because there are so many advantages for both mother and baby (as we've already seen) that most husbands would be hard pushed *not* to be convinced if they knew the whole story. But in addition to this there are positive advantages from their point of view.

While a baby gorilla is being born the father fusses about the mother and when she has given birth he lifts the baby up to her breast at once so that she can suckle it. As we've already seen, this would be difficult for most human fathers to do in the West because of the problems involved in hospital births. But it doesn't mean it's impossible. Once you and your wife have made the decision that she will breast feed your baby and that you will encourage her, you should try and help right from the start.

We feel that even (or indeed especially) at this early stage you the father can take a positive hand in encouraging your baby to feed properly. In some hospitals you'll also have to help your wife beat off attempts made by the hospital staff to give the baby glucose water or bottles of milk. The best thing to do is to tell the sister and the doctor that you both want your baby totally breast fed. You'll find it's best to tell them before the birth, preferably on admission to the maternity unit. A word of warning – don't be fobbed off. Misguided midwives and doctors in some hospitals will try to persuade you that it doesn't matter if the baby has the odd bottle. It's *your* baby, not theirs and it's up to you to hold out for what you feel is right.

If you do discuss this matter with the nursing or medical staff after the birth, make sure that you don't have any scenes in front of your wife as this could upset her and so make breast feeding more difficult.

Having helped your wife get the baby to the breast, stay with her if at all possible. She's just been through the greatest event in her life and will want you there for company and to share in her happiness. We should like to see more hospitals giving a private half hour or so to parents with their new baby so they can both enjoy the experience before the pressures of everyday life impinge on them again.

It's right here in the delivery room that you start looking after your wife in a new way. She may not be able to take in everything that's going on if only because she's so emotionally and physically keyed up. It's an interesting fact that women who have difficult or unpleasant labours tend to be less likely to breast feed. So everything you can do to help your wife, even this early on, will help her breast feed more successfully. In the USA it's common practice to ask the woman if she'd like to breast feed or not immediately after the birth and if the answer is 'no' then she is given an injection to dry up her milk there and then. (In some hospitals they aren't even asked, they simply get the injection!) Of course, most women are in no fit state to make any rational decision about a matter like this in the few minutes after giving birth and undoubtedly many women who would like to have fed their babies will have had their milk suppressed because they didn't want to say 'no' to anything the hospital suggested. This practice is not common in the UK where drugs are now only rarely used to dry up milk but there are parallels and the presence of a 'with it' father can be a great help.

If your wife is going to have problems it's in the first week that they'll be worst. This is unfortunate because it's at this time that so many women are at their lowest and need most help. One experienced breast feeding counsellor has gone so far as to say that successful lactation depends on the woman's helpers and advisers and not on her ability to produce milk. Unfortunately midwives in some hospitals make new mothers feel bad by making them feel like a milk-producing appendage to the baby. Sometimes there is an internal conflict in the mind of the midwife who likes to think of all the babies on the ward as 'hers'.

As soon as the mother shows any signs of having problems with feeding, such midwives jump in with a bottle and so 'take over' the baby. You should ensure that this doesn't happen.

But however useful you may be in the few days your wife spends in hospital, your real help begins when she comes home. If you have other children you'll have been pretty busy looking after them already. Take a couple of weeks off work if you can, so that you can look after the other children and be around when your wife comes home.

Once home, your wife will need you as provider, protector and general helper. For breast feeding to succeed you'll need to play a very important part in the life of the family for the next few weeks. This should be no great hardship – after all most of us only have two children in a lifetime so it should be no problem to give your wife the support and help she'll need during this crucial period.

Most women will come home from hospital and expect to run the house exactly as before. Women tell us that they feel their poor husbands have already been alone with the children long enough and need a rest themselves. If your wife is going to breast feed successfully, don't be under any illusions – she'll need your help. Obviously you'll need to go on providing for her in a material sense but she'll also need a lot of love and emotional back-up.

Apart from providing a happy home environment you'll have to protect her from the children, from well-meaning but ill-informed busy bodies and most of all from herself. Children will be no less demanding now than they were before the baby came and you'll need to keep them amused so that your wife can rest. It's a shame that some babies hardly get to know their mothers because there are so many other people making their own demands on her time. You must act as a buffer between her and the world around her. Relatives and neighbours will be keen to see the baby. Make sure they come in small doses. Many's the time a recently delivered mother gets so exhausted from regaling the world with her hospital sagas that she simply can't relate to or feed her new baby properly.

Breast feeding is a deeply emotional business. Research studies the world over have shown that mammals of many species (and woman is no exception) simply produce less milk or indeed none at all if they are disturbed or stressed while breast feeding. A woman has to become cow-like when feeding her baby, at least in the early weeks until lactation is really well established. Serenity is a must for really successful breast feeding and it's up to you, the husband, to promote it.

Another thing you'll have to provide is encouragement. Studies have shown that women whose husbands don't want them to breast feed rarely manage to do so. Even if the husband is merely 'neutral' the chances of successful feeding are greatly reduced. One American breast feeding counsellor (who guarantees success) will not accept a woman as a client unless her husband approves of breast feeding. So clearly it's best if you show a positive attitude right from the start. It's a lot more difficult to breast feed than to bottle feed in the first few days and your wife will need correspondingly more help which will throw new strains on to you.

To some degree the new dad gets shut out of the excitement of the first few days. The new mother is so closely involved with her baby that he may well feel that the baby is hogging the limelight. Obviously this is true to some extent and it's only fair to let a woman revel in her new baby – but both mother and father have got to get used to a new person with all its physical and emotional demands and that's never easy. We're not suggesting for a moment that poor dad should become a pitiable figure that lurks in the shadows. On the contrary, although he'll have to do more than usual it should be a wonderful time for both parents.

The majority of women are highly emotional after having a baby – their hormones keep them keyed up to respond to their babies. But as well as reacting to their baby's every whimper they may also react to the world around them in a way which is atypical for them. Even the toughest professional woman who holds down a big job in everyday life may well collapse in tears for no apparent reason. Sometimes she'll do this because she's happy and this is very often difficult for a man to understand.

Just a little word of warning. Do be careful about what you say.

Your wife will often be so dependent on you that almost anything you say might upset her. This is especially true when discussing breast feeding. Husbands play a vital role in whether their wives carry on breast feeding or not and often a casual, thoughtless remark can throw a woman completely off and make her feel inadequate. Until breast feeding is well and truly established be very sensitive about what you say!

Two of the things that worry husbands most about breast feeding (or at least the two things they most often talk about which isn't necessarily the same thing at all) are whether their wives will (a) go off sex and (b) lose their figures. The next chapter is all about sex and breast feeding so more of that later but here let's look at the figure question. Whether most of the breast feeding experts like it or not, men today think of breasts first and foremost as sexual objects. We get rather tired of the 'experts' who keep telling us that breasts are functional organs for feeding babies. Of course they are but not exclusively so and for the forty-odd years of the average couple's married life their erotic role is vastly more important. It seems ridiculous to pretend that husbands' fears about their wives having droopy breasts after feeding are unjustified.

All breasts enlarge during pregnancy regardless of whether the woman is going to breast feed or not but if she does feed her baby, her breasts will be bigger for longer. Strange as it may seem, the research into breast size after breast feeding is scanty and confused. But overall one thing does emerge. Women who had breast fed for two weeks or more reported that their breasts had become slightly droopier. They also felt that overall the pleasure they had from feeding their babies far outweighed this slight loss of figure. Had they known the medical arguments for breast feeding they would without a doubt have been even less concerned about the long-term effects on their breasts than they were.

But does this slight deterioration really matter? Did you, you should ask yourself, marry your wife simply for her breasts? And how many women that you see walking around who've had children have such unpleasant breasts that you don't want to look at them? The quest for perfect breasts is not only a little crazy but it's also thoroughly unrealistic because most of us don't marry girls out of the centre spread of *Playboy* in the first place. Breasts quite naturally change with age and breast feeding might just hasten this change a little, if at all.

A lot of fathers tell us that they quite like the idea of their wives breast feeding but feel it leaves them with little they can do for the baby. If that's the case it's a shame because having a baby is a joint affair and enjoying it should be too. It's helpful to remember that babies aren't like dogs – they don't go in for cupboard love. Whether you give the baby the odd feed or two is really beside the point. Any father who thinks he'll get nothing positive out of his child being breast fed should think again because there are lots of ways that he'll benefit.

First, he'll never have to get up at night to prepare a feed and that's no mean advantage when he's at work again. The family can't run out of milk powder at awkward times either. Breast feeding does make extra demands on the mother's body and so she has to eat more than normal, but even allowing for the cost of these extra calories breast feeding is still less expensive than formula feeding according to three major studies. But whatever artificial milk costs it's one thing less you'll have to remember to buy and means there are fewer baby things to carry when you go out anywhere. As this usually falls on you that's another big advantage.

Last of all and probably most important is the pleasure it'll give you. You'll get this by seeing your wife happy, content and fulfilled by being a real 'female' mother. Many women revel in this feeling of femininity and their husbands often benefit from it too.

But there are still many husbands who feel they won't have as much fun with and won't be as close to their new baby as they would have been if they had been helping with the bottle feeding. This is a sad argument because there are lots of other things a father can do – he can cuddle his baby, play with him, bath and change him and even babysit sometimes so that his wife can get out alone if only for half an hour to see a friend or neighbour. A little time on her own can give the nursing mother a great boost and it's well worth planning the odd outing so that your wife has something to look forward to. Don't get carried away, though, with the idea of her going off on her own because whenever she does this it'll have to be timed around the baby's feeds.

You may feel that we've made it all sound rather hard going for the new breast feeding dad! If we have, it's only to point out some of the ways in which you can help your wife do something that'll bring pleasure to you both and give your baby the best start he could get in life. Just think of all the time and money you're going to lavish on your children over the years yet so many husbands seem to cheeseparé their time and affection in the first vital weeks. If you do help your wife, it'll really make a big difference.

15 Breast feeding and sex

In all the books, learned medical papers and popular magazine articles that have been written about breast feeding, few say much (if anything) about breast feeding as a sexual experience. Yet the deep-seated sexual nature of breast feeding is only too apparent to many nursing mothers. The trouble is that we live in a repressed society even in this so-called 'permissive age' and many women feel guilty linking sexual pleasure with breast feeding. If they experience anything more than a 'pleasant' feeling they are uneasy and often intensely guilty because 'everyone knows that no one but your husband should arouse feelings like that'. It's because this guilt and other sexual hangups are such common causes for the failure of breast feeding that we've devoted a whole chapter to the subject.

When you think about it, breast feeding, like intercourse, must have been pleasurable throughout history or Man would never have kept going as successfully as he has! If there were two things that had to be pleasant to ensure the continuance of the species, sex and breast feeding were the ones.

This link between sexual pleasure and breast feeding comes as a bolt from the blue for many women and even positively revolts some. A psychiatrist with a special knowledge of this subject made a television broadcast recently in which he suggested that some women actually had orgasms when breast feeding – a well-documented occurrence although by no means a common one. The switchboard was jammed with outraged women, one of whom phoned to say she had actually vomited while he was talking. It's this sort of attitude, though of course it's usually severely repressed, that makes a lot of women either not breast feed at all or fail when they do. Feelings of sexuality are only acceptable to most of us within certain very strict bounds – and breast feeding a baby comes outside them!

To see why this is contrary to what Nature intended and why such Victorian taboos hinder breast feeding a century later, let's look at some basic and undeniable facts. To a man, sex means intercourse. If he is making love to the woman he loves and who is the mother of his children – so much the better. But often men will say how readily they can enjoy intercourse with a woman who means little or nothing to them. Men are relatively simple in their sexual demands and relatively easily pleased.

To a woman, on the other hand, sex means much more. True, some women are like men and can centre their sex lives on their orgasms but this is uncommon. To most women sexuality is a much more complex and enduring thing, and often a more emotional business than it is for a man. A woman's sexuality begins in earnest in her teens and soon she is on her way to looking for a loving, considerate sex partner and possibly a father for her potential children. As if all this weren't enough, her sexuality takes an even more fulfilling and dramatic turn when she becomes pregnant and carries a baby around inside her for several months. Her body changes in numerous ways – as does her mind – and many experts say that she'll never feel the same again because she's felt something she's never experienced before and her relationship with her child gives her a new outlook on life and herself.

At the end of pregnancy she gives birth to a baby – another remarkable physical and emotional experience – and then feeds it. Or does she?

Primitive women were ruled by their cycles. Breast feeding did, and still does, perform a more important role as a contraceptive than all the man-made methods put together – indeed, this is how families are spaced by most solely breast feeding peoples. Many millions of women the world over are either pregnant or lactating for the whole of their reproductive lives and are ruled by their hormones from the age of twelve until the menopause.

Today's woman doesn't want to be ruled by her hormones and social changes have made her loath to have babies every two or three years, spaced only by her breast feeding contraception. Today's woman wants to be more like a man than ever before and society does everything possible to ensure that this happens. This move started in earnest in the 1920s when women began to become an important economic force in the country and union leaders, industrialists and parents today all agree that life is becoming so expensive in the Western world that it is scarcely possible for one breadwinner per family to cope. Indeed, many industries now depend on female labour and the country would probably grind to a halt if they were not in the work force. More than half of all the married women in this country work.

Women have therefore become geared up to expect more education, to work for at least a part of their lives, to put off getting married and having children and generally to try – often against their will, it's true – to be more like men. And we're not just talking about women's libbers. This attitude is now common in almost every stratum of society. Whereas professional and highly skilled women used to be the only ones in this group, it now includes office, factory and shop girls. A survey of American women showed that given the choice, 25 per cent of them would like to be reborn as men whilst only 3 per cent of men said they'd like to be reborn as women.

All right, we can hear you say. That's all very well but women are equal to men and so deserve equal opportunity. True. But one way in which they're very *different* from men is in their hormones. Modern society has tried to make women the same as men when their whole physiological make-up is different and whether we like it or not we are still ruled by the basic laws of Nature. If we ignore these laws we must expect to pay the price. It's because modern women are by and large loath to be *female* any more (although they are probably more *feminine* than ever) that breast feeding has declined in popularity. Breast feeding makes a woman realize that she really is a *woman* and that isn't very fashionable today as we've just seen. What makes her a *woman* is her hormones.

Once you understand how a woman's whole make-up revolves around her hormones, you'll be in a much better position to understand how to make breast feeding successful in today's society and also to see how closely it's linked with sex.

Although most people don't realize it, there's a tremendous similarity between a woman's periods, pregnancies, orgasms and lactation. During all of these her breasts become bigger for a start. Most women also feel protective or 'motherly' after intercourse, after giving birth and during breast feeding. This is no accident and stems from the fact that a woman's sex hormones act on several parts of her body at once and in different situations. For instance, oxytocin, the hormone that we've seen to be so crucial for the let-down reflex, is also released during orgasm and at birth.

However much we choose to deny it, a woman's sexuality is often linked to a feeling of motherliness. Today, though, it's only fashionable to stress the mechanics of sex and, as a result, magazine articles abound with hints on achieving the perfect orgasm and attaining ninety-five different love positions. We feel sure that this quest for perfect orgasms (and preferably plenty of them) is a subconscious substitute for many of the other *female* joys that so many women now get either not at all, or very late in life (in biological terms).

Today, a woman's breasts have taken on a far more important role in the eyes of most people – a sexual one. Breasts have become the erotic focus for most Western men and are now an integral part of the fabric of modern society. When did you last see a gorgeous foot advertising a new cigar? No one knows why certain societies 'home in' on a particular part of the female anatomy in this way but it's interesting that man is the only mammal in which the female's breasts develop before they're actually needed to feed the young. There's no reason to suppose, though, that it's because of this that they have taken on an erotic role; in fact, we in the West are unusual among our fellow men in placing such erotic value on the breast.

So, with men putting such a sexual emphasis on the breast, is it surprising that sexual overtones often mitigate very strongly against breast feeding? Studies show that many women won't even consider breast feeding simply because they believe it will ruin their breasts and so make them less sexually attractive. If you find this difficult to believe, bear in mind that just about the commonest subject on which agony columnists in the women's press receive letters is that of breast size and you'll soon see that there really is a problem.

Many women get sexual pleasure from breast stimulation by their partners and studies show that some women can actually experience orgasm from breast stimulation alone. This is scarcely surprising as the clitoris, uterus and nipples are interconnected by nerves in certain parts of the brain. So not only do women's hormones (mostly oxytocin) link these organs but her nervous pathways do too.

Let's look first at the sexual feelings a woman gets when breast feeding. For women who relate easily to their bodies, breast feeding is often a highly pleasurable experience. For them, at worst it's a pleasant, relaxing way of feeding a baby but at best it's a highly stimulating event which frankly 'turns them on'. All shades in between are completely normal and by definition most women will fall somewhere between the two. Replies to doctors who ask the right questions show that many breast feeding women feel sexually aroused albeit in a controlled and simple way. Many notice some vaginal lubrication and a few even actually have an orgasm. We get the impression that breast feeding engenders more positively enjoyable feelings in women than they will admit – even to themselves. Whilst most women certainly do not have orgasms, very many do describe a powerful parallel experience which is less explosive and more calming. They also get a feeling of euphoria or wellbeing after a feed which is much like that after an orgasm.

Many women say that they find breast feeding so sexually pleasing that they feel more sexy towards their husbands. In fact, it's well known that women who are nursing return to sexual intercourse sooner after birth than do their bottle feeding sisters. Certainly the breast feeding woman returns to normal more quickly physically but it's also likely that the repeated feelings of sexual arousal (however minimal they are) also make her more receptive to sex. Some studies show that a substantial number of women are more sexually active when breast feeding than at any other time. This is good news for fathers who often feel left out at this time!

But if a woman gets pleasure from having her baby stimulate, play with and feed from her breasts, her husband may well not enjoy the baby's relationship with his wife. Until now, his wife's breasts have 'belonged' to him and he may resent the little intruder. As we've already mentioned, a husband can actually put a woman off feeding successfully simply by being negative – but he shouldn't be blamed. So many things make him think of her breasts as erotic that it's hardly surprising that he'll feel bad about somebody usurping his role, especially since that somebody is now taking up most of her time and love.

The thing is to be positive. Show your husband you still love and want him. Don't let him feel that because the baby's feeding, that's all you see your breasts as doing. Let your husband play with your breasts as he did before. He can even drink your milk if he wants to; he won't be robbing the baby of anything because, as we've seen, the more milk your breasts are asked to produce, the more they will produce. Should you feel sexually aroused by breast feeding, this can be pleasant for your partner too. One woman we know found breast feeding too demanding because she felt so sexy she wore her husband out! This brings us to the negative side of the whole story because these pleasant feelings make some women feel guilty.

Most women are shy of their breasts. Strange though it may seem in an age where breasts assault us from all sides, women are very insecure about them. Men look at beautiful girls because they get a simple animal pleasure from them – women look at them to see what other women have that they haven't. And usually it's breasts they're comparing. If society encouraged topless bathing, naturist beaches and open display of the breasts in fashion, then perhaps women would not feel so shy. The fact is, they still do. It's this feeling of shyness, propriety and frank prudery that puts many women off starting to breast feed. Little do they know that a hormonally induced change takes place in breast feeding mothers that enables them to feed in public with equanimity. They wouldn't have dreamt of baring their breasts in public before the baby was born and won't after they've stopped breast feeding either!

But even if most women could overcome this aversion to

showing their breasts, a substantial proportion simply don't like their breasts touched or played with even by their partners – let alone by a champing baby. Kinsey found that up to 50 per cent of all non-pregnant women found breast stimulation unpleasant or sexually unarousing. In such cases there's precious little a book like this can do. Indeed, we know some women who are completely revolted by the whole idea of suckling a baby at all and it's nearly impossible to convince them that it will be pleasant. Only another woman who once felt the same way but later changed her mind can do that.

Breast feeding succeeds best in breast-orientated *female* women who like their breasts and like having them touched. A study in the USA found that women who failed to breast feed had substantially more sexual hangups than those who succeeded. Another piece of research showed that 65 per cent of women who successfully breast fed 'positively enjoyed the experience', but that still left 35 per cent who didn't! Most of these found it unpleasant because they thought it 'immodest' and 'distasteful'.

For most women, the comparison with cows doesn't go unnoticed and in today's so-called sophisticated society this can be a considerable turn-off. It really isn't an unreasonable comparison, though, because lactating women *are* like cows if they are lactating cows! So what, though – cows also walk around in fields yet that doesn't stop us going for country walks.

Some women actually become less sexy when breast feeding. For them, the tenderness of their breasts (especially a long time after a feed) makes breast play painful and this can turn them off sex. The way round this is to breast feed before sexual intercourse. Some women point out that their nipples don't erect as much as they used to and that they lose sexual pleasure because of this. This is in fact an illusion. The nipples do erect in a lactating woman but their increase in size can be masked by the already swollen breast. It's the same with breast size. Some women get pleasure from the swelling of their breasts when they're stimulated during sex play. The lactating breast doesn't swell (because it's already so big) and this can make the woman feel that she's not responding in the usual way.

Some couples find that the woman's breasts get in the way or are painful in certain love-making positions. This can easily be overcome by changing to another position and anyway is only a problem for about the first two months. Another problem is that during intense sexual excitement milk may spurt or leak from your nipples. This can be exciting for the man but some people don't like it simply because it can be so messy. If this upsets you or your partner, try feeding the baby before you make love and this will reduce the likelihood of spurting.

The foundation stones of successful breast feeding are laid early on in a couple's married life. Whilst it's by no means a common subject of honeymoon conversation, the more a man plays with his wife's breasts, stimulates them and makes sure she likes it, the better the chances that she will even consider breast feeding when the time comes. Remember, the size and shape of your breasts and nipples have no bearing on the enjoyment you and your husband will get from them – and this goes for baby too.

During pregnancy we suggest that the only nipple care that should take place at all for normal nipples is that carried out by your husband. Get him to roll them gently between his fingers or in his mouth during love play. You don't need, or indeed want, doctors or midwives doing anything.

Breast feeding itself shouldn't interfere with sexual intercourse – and it had better not because you'll be breast feeding for at least four months and probably much longer if you want to. Any husband who gives the ultimatum 'baby or me' is doing all three of you a great disfavour. If you really feel strongly about feeding your baby even though it's at a very late stage, try and persuade your husband. You certainly won't do this by 'going off' him so *share your breasts with him and the baby*.

Childbirth and especially the birth of the first child is a big upheaval for your husband. If anything, it's easier for you because you've got all the joys (and otherwise!) of looking after the baby. Your husband is often only an interested bystander.

Finally, here are a few hints on how to combine a good sex life with a happy breast feeding baby.

1 Make sure your husband doesn't feel left out – physically or emotionally.

2 If feeding makes you feel sexy or even simply pleasantly relaxed, tell him so to encourage him to make the most of it.

3 Wear a good nursing bra and remind him you're doing it for his benefit so that he'll have your breasts looking good years from now.

4 Respect his wishes not to feed in public or in front of certain people if you know it upsets him.

5 Plan the odd trip out together once your let-down is well established. Express some breast milk and leave it for the baby sitter to give. You can't expect your husband to look favourably on breast feeding if he thinks he's going to be tied to the house for the next six months.

6 Keep up your previous 'mistress' image as much as possible.

16 Feeding the older baby

Weaning

Weaning means different things to different people but we define it as taking a baby off breast milk and feeding him with other sources of nourishment. When, how and why you wean are entirely up to you, though we think it's important to discuss some important points, including the foods you give your baby to replace your breast milk.

When should you wean?

Take no notice of the various pamphlets and baby books you read which give you precise instructions as to the exact age or weight your baby should be when you start weaning. There is no such age or weight and there should be no hard and fast rules.

As long as your baby is thriving, happy and gaining weight regularly and as long as you are both enjoying it, carry on breast feeding him.

It's easier to say when you shouldn't start weaning! Breast milk alone is the best food for your baby for at least the first four months and for longer if he is satisfied. If you introduce cows' milk and solids before four months you are not only laying yourself open to the possibility of reducing your milk supply, but you are also laying your baby open to the chance of foreign protein leaking into his bloodstream via his gut lining and possibly causing sensitization if he is susceptible. This, as we've seen, may lead to the development of allergies.

There are two ways of introducing other foods – either you can wait until your baby shows a real interest in the food the rest of the family is eating, and let him pick up some of this food with his fingers, or you can give him spoonfuls of food if he shows no particular interest. The first way would seem to be the most sensible, though if left to themselves some babies might carry on with breast milk alone for rather longer than would seem nutritionally advisable.

If it's left to the baby to decide when he wants to start finger feeding, he'll probably try at about six months or so. As this is also the age at which many babies get their first tooth, it seems likely that this is the age Nature intended babies to start on foods other than breast milk.

There's no need to offer him spoonfuls of food before six to eight months if he's thriving, as breast milk will provide adequate amounts of all nutrients for the majority of babies till then. Later in the second half of the first year your baby will need more than breast milk alone can provide, though there is no need to give large amounts of food straight away – increase it slowly as he wants it.

One exception to this general rule is the premature baby whose liver stores of iron may not be large enough to last for six months until other foods are introduced. Iron is stored in the baby's liver in the last few weeks of pregnancy in particular, so if the baby is born early, he may not have enough iron to last for six months on milk alone. It's an easy enough matter for your doctor to test a drop of your baby's blood to see if there is any danger of anaemia developing, so it's worth while asking for this test (though it will probably be suggested anyway) at least once in the first six months.

Iron supplements can be given if necessary, though in practice they rarely are necessary for the fully breast fed baby. It's a fact that premature bottle fed babies are more likely to become anaemic than premature breast fed babies, even though the level of iron in modified cows' milk is higher than that in breast milk. This is because breast milk iron is better absorbed than cows' milk iron.

Once you have introduced other foods, you can carry on breast feeding as long as your baby wants and as long as your milk supply lasts. Some mothers find their babies lose interest in the breast relatively soon while others find their babies don't seem to want to give it up at all. The milk supply should last as long as you want it to if you are giving your baby virtually all his fluid in this way. If you give him other drinks and only one or two breast feeds a day, your milk will slowly dry up, though some mothers manage to retain a single feed for many months and find it's a sure way of helping their babies settle down at night.

There is no hard and fast rule of how long lactation should last. As long as the baby is stimulating your breasts, they'll produce milk. Wet nurses used to carry on feeding for years on end and many mothers the world over feed their children for several years. The Western idea that milk automatically dries up after a few months is totally wrong.

What are the advantages of carrying on breast feeding after six months? First, your baby will continue to receive protection against infection though full breast feeding only gives this advantage for eight months, after which time, from the infection point of view, your baby is just as well off without your milk. In fact, babies fully breast fed (with no additional food) for longer than eight months are at greater risk from infection than babies who are being weaned by then, so this is one argument for introducing solids by eight months.

Second, you and your baby probably enjoy feed times together and will be extremely disappointed to give them up. Breast feeding offers your baby emotional as well as nutritional sustenance – an older baby often turns to the breast to find comfort when he is upset. Many mothers remember their very real feeling of loss when they gave their baby his last breast feed and they also remember their anguish at the tears and frustration of the baby denied the breast because it was felt to be the 'right' time to wean. There is no need for anguish either on your part or your baby's. *Simply let him decide when he wants to stop feeding and go along with him. This is what is known as 'baby-led' weaning*. Whether he gives up the breast at nine months or eighteen, or even later, by doing it alone he'll be happier than if you make him give it up.

So, the answer to the question when to wean is not as simple as you might have thought. Solids should be introduced not earlier than four months and not later than eight months but breast feeding can continue for as long as you and your baby both want it too.

How to stop breast feeding

If you have to stop breast feeding for some reason, it's far easier for you to do it gradually, almost without thinking about it. If you try and stop quickly, you'll probably end up with a fractious baby and painful, engorged breasts. There is no place for drying-up pills today – they have certain unpleasant side-effects, and are unnecessary anyway.

Give up the feed at which you have least milk first. This is usually the one in the late afternoon or early evening. Give your baby something else to drink instead: some mothers have strong feelings against bottles and make their babies drink from a cup as soon as they start weaning. If you have to wean, it's worth remembering that babies enjoy sucking and a bottle may be more enjoyable for him than a cup. If you're weaning later and intend letting your baby breast feed when he wants to for comfort, if not for milk, then give him his drink from a cup.

After a week or so, give up another breast feed and carry on in this way until you are only feeding once a day. You may find that it is most comfortable to give up the early morning feed last, as you'll probably have most milk at this feed. Some mothers like to give up the last feed of the day last of all, as their babies seem to enjoy this the most and sleep well afterwards.

Weaning should be unhurried and unworried. Certainly if you can possibly avoid it, don't ever wean in an emergency – there is almost always a way round the problem. Your baby would find it very hard to understand why he was suddenly denied the breast and might be upset for some time.

If your baby asks for a feed by nuzzling against your breast several days after you have stopped feeding him, let him feed. He'll soon realize that there is little, if any, milk there, though he may want to suck for comfort if not for food.

What should I give my baby to eat?

If your baby's first foods are 'finger foods' – foods that he can pick up himself with his hands and suck on or bite, then the choice of food is great. Let him have any raw fruit such as a large piece of apple or banana; a rusk of baked wholemeal bread; in fact anything hard that won't be likely to break into pieces and choke him. He'll eat it by gradually dissolving it in his mouth.

If you're starting off with spoonfuls of food, remember that at first he won't be able to chew anything, so the food must be soft enough to swallow.

Whatever the method of feeding, the basic principles behind a healthy diet for your baby are the same. He'll do best on a balanced diet containing protein, fat, carbohydrate, minerals and vitamins, though at first of course he'll still be getting most of his food from your milk, so you needn't worry about giving him a balance of these nutrients until breast milk plays a less important role in his diet.

Some important points to realize are that it is quite unnecessary for a baby (or indeed anyone) to eat any added sugar. Sugar rots the teeth and makes people fat without contributing anything worthwhile to the diet. Natural sugar in fruit and vegetables will taste quite sweet enough to your baby and if you can help him grow up without a sweet tooth you'll be doing him a great favour. Similarly, it's far better to give your baby unrefined carbohydrates – there is no need for him to have white, refined flour in any form, be it in cakes, biscuits, bread or puddings. Cook with wholemeal flour and you'll be standing him in good stead for the future. A diet high in unrefined carbohydrates will help protect a person from bowel disease among others for the rest of his life. A baby brought up on a diet which contains unrefined carbohydrate (rich in dietary fibre) and very little sugar will also be unlikely to get fat, which is another plus point.

Another thing best avoided is salt. Salt can actually be dangerous for a young baby if given in excess. It's worth remembering that your older baby will enjoy his food just as much without salt added and he will lose nothing by not having it.

Today's consumer society buys vast amounts of packaged, processed foods which bear little resemblance to their natural state. Colourings, flavourings, emulsifiers, stabilizers, bleaches and many other chemicals are added to these foods and the public buys them with delight as many are so easy to prepare and look so bright and cheerful. Ideally, it would be better if you only gave your baby 'natural foods', without any commercial interference in the way of food additives. Although there is legislation regulating the use of these chemicals, many legal additives have recently come under the suspicion of being harmful. What is more, some are banned in some countries but not in others. Much more research is necessary before certain additives can be pronounced truly safe, so you and your family are better off avoiding them.

There's no need to use tinned or dried baby foods – simply give your baby whatever you are going to eat, mashed or sieved first.

If you live in an area with low levels of fluoride in the drinking water, you may want to give the baby fluoride supplements in the form of tablets or drops. Ask your dentist about the local water and the amount of fluoride you should be giving. Fluoride cuts tooth decay by half.

One question frequently asked is whether a baby needs cows' milk once he's weaned from the breast. The answer is no. There is nothing in cows' milk which he can't get from other food sources, providing he has a balanced diet. Even if he had no cheese or butter he would still be all right. If he likes milk, though, let him drink it.

As we live in a relatively sunless climate, many doctors advise giving pre-school children extra Vitamin D as a daily supplement. Vitamin D is normally formed in the skin by the action of sunlight but it is possible to become deficient if shut indoors all day. Vitamin C is often included with Vitamin D supplements which is just as well because so many mothers destroy dietary Vitamin C by cooking their food too long. Be careful to give only the recommended amounts of Vitamin D as it's harmful to give too much.

What drinks should your baby have to replace your milk? As we've said, he doesn't have to have cows' milk. The most popular drink for young children seems to be orange or blackcurrant syrup diluted with water. These syrups or squashes contain a lot of sugar, often with other additives such as colourings and flavourings, and are highly likely to cause tooth decay. While some of these drinks do contain Vitamin C (one of the reasons mothers have for giving them) not all do and many contain no natural fruit juice at all. Your baby will do very well if you only give him water to drink. If you want to give something else, give him the juice of a sweet orange diluted with water, or fresh orange juice.

Can you breast feed while you are having a period?
The answer is yes. There is no reason why you shouldn't as it won't harm you or the baby. Some mothers say that their babies are rather fractious around period time. This is quite likely to be due to their own pre-menstrual tension being communicated to their babies, rather than to any difference in the milk. Some babies do have diarrhoea for a couple of days though.

Can you breast feed if you are pregnant?
You can breast feed right through a pregnancy if you want to and if your milk supply lasts in spite of the pregnancy hormones. Indeed, in some parts of the world a mother will carry on feeding her toddler along with the new baby. This can present problems if the toddler is allowed first call on the breast, as the baby may not get enough to drink, especially if the mother herself is undernourished. In some developing countries, though, weaning the older child would be even more hazardous than allowing both to breast feed, as there is often not enough food for the family and the toddler might easily become undernourished without his breast milk.

Some mothers find that their breast milk tends to diminish during pregnancy. This is probably because the circulating pregnancy hormones affect milk production. The milk, however, changes in quality to become richer in fats and vitamins, so is in no way inferior even though its volume may be less.

Once again we see that the way to manage natural breast feeding is to do away with any rules and regulations, and to be led as far as possible by your own baby and by your common sense. Let breast feeding your baby be followed by baby-led weaning if you possibly can – you'll both find it easier.

Breast feeding the older child
In this country the vast majority of breast fed babies are weaned

from the breast by a year but there is no reason why you should do this if you don't want to. An increasing number of mothers are feeding for longer periods – some until their children are two, three or even older.

Breast feeding the older child is more important for the psychological comfort and pleasure it gives rather than for the nutritional value which is by then supplied, in most cases in the Western world at least, by other foods. There is often little pattern to the feeds – the child comes for a drink when he feels like cuddling and being close to his mother, perhaps when he is upset or tired.

You may well notice a difficult patch between four and six months when you wonder whether you really want to go on feeding. You'll feel this way for several reasons. First, you're feeling so much better in yourself that you want to get going again in the outside world; second, your baby will be more demanding, more aware and may cry more; third, he may be demanding more to eat and so make you feel you haven't got enough milk. Lastly, you may be feeling that breast feeding is going to go on for ever and so may be becoming disenchanted with it.

Don't get dispirited. If you feel you've had enough of breast feeding, give it up gradually as we've suggested. It's better that you stop and carry on developing a loving relationship with your baby than start to resent feeding him.

If you carry on feeding as your baby passes the year stage, your only problem will be coping with uncalled-for and often unkind criticism from friends, neighbours and relatives. Many of them will be surprised that you actually want to go on doing it for so long after other mothers have stopped! This sort of criticism can be very off-putting but if you and your baby want to go on, it's really none of their business.

To spare their amazement and your embarrassment, you may find it a good idea to feed your older baby alone. It's scarcely surprising that a society which finds it hard to cope with the sight of a little baby being breast fed finds it even more difficult to cope with an older breast fed child. If your child tugs at your clothes or actually asks for a feed when you are out visiting, make some excuse and go into another room to feed him. Don't make him feel there is anything shameful in what you are doing and don't feel ashamed yourself either!

However long you feed your baby (provided you do so for at least four to six months) you'll know you've done the best thing for him and will almost certainly have enjoyed it yourself. Just how long you go on for is very much a matter of personal choice – there are no rules and no known medical benefits after about eight months. Don't let this put you off going on for longer, though, because breast feeding is an invaluable part of being a good mother and whatever the experts say and however many fads come and go, good mothering will always be at the heart of happy family life.

17 Readers' questions and answers

Introduction

In the three years since we wrote *Breast is Best* there has been a flood of research reports, letters to the medical and nursing journals and editorials in the learned scientific and medical press about breast feeding. In fact, breast feeding has become very much an 'in' subject both in the eyes of mothers and the medical profession.

Although many of the learned papers have been concerned with scientific matters, others have centred on the benefits of demand feeding and uninterrupted contact between a mother and her baby. There have been no suggestions that restricted or schedule feeding is desirable or successful.

Some health professionals expressed annoyance over parts of the book they took to be critical of them. However, many of them have taken such criticisms as a challenge and are redoubling their efforts to work with mothers to increase the numbers of successful breast feeders. The next set of figures for breast feeding mothers will undoubtedly show a considerable improvement on current ones.

Because of all this interest and because *Breast is Best* has created an enormous number of enquiries, we decided to update it. This new section contains information about the most recent research and effectively brings *Breast is Best* right up to date for the 1980s.

In 1974, the UK Department of Health recommended that mothers should be encouraged to breast feed their babies for at least the first two weeks of life, but preferably for four to six months. They also concluded that, for most babies, milk alone is adequate for normal growth and development during the first four to six months of life.

The Working Party of the Panel of Child Nutrition which wrote the report realized that there was a lack of up-to-date information on infant feeding practices on a national scale. To remedy this a national survey of over 2,000 babies was undertaken by the Office of Population Censuses and Surveys (OPCS) in 1975, and this provided a representative sample of all births during a period of one month in England and Wales. The results of this Report were not available until after the first edition of *Breast is Best* was in press so here we'll give some of the more important findings.

The information in the report of the survey holds lessons for us all. First, it underlines very strongly the fact that in England and Wales in 1975 at least, *bottle feeding was the norm.* To be fair though, the recommendations made in 1974 had had relatively little time to take effect. The following table is made up from figures given in the OPCS report.

Percentage of women breast or bottle feeding at different periods after birth

	breast feeding (%)		*bottle feeding* (%)
Birth	51		46
	fully	*partially*	
Two weeks	14	35	51
Six weeks	4	24	72
Four months	<1	13	86
Six months	0	9	91

We can see from this table that although about one in two mothers starts to breast feed her baby after the birth, less than one in four of these mothers is still fully breast feeding her baby at two weeks. The figures kept by maternity units for the percentage of mothers breast feeding on leaving hospital can look unduly rosy unless they are broken down into the percentage of mothers fully breast feeding, and the percentage partially breast feeding (giving cows' milk complements). Although a mother whose baby is having complements *can* increase her milk supply and wean her baby from cows' milk, this requires more expert advice from health professionals and more knowledge of the physiology of lactation and confidence on her part than is usually available. It's virtually true to say that by two weeks, three out of four breast feeding mothers in this survey were already on the way to full bottle feeding.

By six weeks, only one in two of the breast feeders was even partially breast feeding. By four months, less than one mother in a hundred was fully breast feeding, and only one in four of the original breast feeders was giving her baby any breast milk at all.

Another interesting fact that emerged from the report was that only 14 per cent of breast-fed babies had *no* cows' milk in the first week. No one could argue that anything like 86 per cent of breast-fed babies *needs* cows' milk, so a lot of babies must have been given it unnecessarily.

It's tempting to assume that the breast feeding statistics were so low because the mothers who started breast feeding wanted to give it up much sooner than experts recommend. However, another table shows that this simply isn't the case. The vast majority of mothers who stop breast feeding are not doing so from choice.

Main reason given by mothers for stopping breast feeding

	stopped by 6 weeks	*stopped between 6 weeks and 4 months*	*stopped between 4 and 6 months*
	%	%	%
Insufficient milk	54	66	38
Painful breasts or nipples	12	4	6
Baby wouldn't suck/ rejected the breast	9	4	11
Inverted nipples	6	–	–
Mother ill	5	9	3
Baby ill	2	3	4
Had breast fed long enough/as long as planned	1	5	25
Breast feeding too tiring/taking too long	1	1	1

Domestic reasons	2	1	5
Embarrassment	2	1	–
Baby can't be fed by others	1	1	–
Didn't like breast feeding	2	–	–
Going back to work	0	3	–
Other reasons	3	2	7
	100	100	100

(from *Infant Feeding 1975; Attitudes and Practice in England and Wales* HMSO SS1064)

The message that comes across from this table is that whatever age the baby is when the mother stops breast feeding, by far the most likely reason for her stopping is an insufficiency of milk. This is more important than nipple soreness, far more important than the almost mythical 'going back to work', and beats breast feeding being 'too tiring' by a long way. Drying up of milk is the main disorder of breast feeding in England and Wales, not to mention the rest of the western, and increasingly the third, world.

The fact that often escapes both mothers and health professionals alike is that an insufficient milk supply is a preventable problem in almost every mother. Just think how much bitter disappointment could be saved if only this were understood.

What advice were these mothers with insufficient milk given before they finally stopped breast feeding altogether? Amazingly, 94 per cent of them were told by their midwife, health visitor or doctor to give cows' milk complements or to stop breast feeding altogether and to put their babies on the bottle. No mention of increasing the milk supply was made except to the lucky 6 per cent, though such advice should have been given straight away. (Unless, of course, a baby was actually ill because of a lack of breast milk, in which case cows' milk or donated milk, should be used while the mother is encouraged to increase her own milk supply.)

Two more tables from the study bring out interesting points.

Reasons given by mothers of first babies for choosing to breast feed

	%
Breast feeding is best for the baby's health	83
Breast feeding is natural	39
Convenience (no bottles to make up or sterilize)	38
Emotional satisfaction (closer relationship between mother and baby)	20
Influenced by friends or relatives	20
Influenced/advised by health personnel	18
Cheaper	17
Helps mother to get her figure back	8
Can't overfeed the baby	8
Don't know/no particular reason	3
Other reasons	4

(percentages do not add to 100 as some mothers gave more than one reason)

(from Infant Feeding 1975: Attitudes and Practice in England and Wales HMSO SS1064)

Reasons given by mothers of first babies for choosing to bottle feed

Don't need privacy for bottle feeding/would be embarrassed to breast feed in front of others	43
Not tied to the baby because others can feed it	38
Don't like the idea of breast feeding	25
Put off breast feeding by experiences of others	17
You know how much milk the baby has had/don't need to worry whether he's had enough	14
Can't breast feed for medical reasons/ advised to bottle feed by health professionals	9
Expecting to return to work soon	6
Don't know/no particular reason	5
Other reasons	7

(percentages do not add to 100 as some mothers gave more than one reason)

The fascinating thing that emerges from these tables is that the mothers who choose to bottle feed all gave negative reasons *against* breast feeding, rather than positive ones *for* bottle feeding. The breast feeders, however, gave positive reasons for breast feeding. Thorough discussion of the imagined disadvantages of breast feeding in antenatal classes, preferably with the help of a mother who is breast feeding successfully, might go a long way to help some of these 'negative' mothers choose breast feeding instead. Also, as the breast feeders give the reason that breast feeding is best for the baby's health as their number one choice, this must obviously be aired well and not hushed up for the sake of allaying guilt on the part of those who don't want to, or really can't breast feed.

Before we leave the report, it's interesting that of the mothers who went to antenatal classes, over a third reported that feeding was not discussed at all. Of those classes which included talks or discussions on infant feeding, only two thirds of the mothers thought that the person running the class had been in favour of breast feeding. These mothers were more likely to plan to breast feed than those mothers who thought no preference had been expressed. It's obvious from this that people running classes should not only include a talk about infant feeding but should also encourage breast feeding.

Drugs and breast feeding

By far the commonest queries we have had since the publication of *Breast is Best* have been on the subject of drugs and breast feeding. The following list includes up-to-date information, more details of the drugs already discussed on pages 165–7 and data on drugs taken by the mother reported to cause any side effects, however mild, in the breast-fed baby. If a drug or drug group is not mentioned, either no breast feeding studies have been done on it or studies have shown that it is safe and has no side-effects.

Side-effects of maternal drugs in the breast-fed baby

Anti-infective drugs

Chloramphenicol May harm bone marrow. May also cause refusal of the breast, sleepiness during feeds and vomiting after. Probably contra-indicated while breast feeding.

Sulphonamides Not absolutely contra-indicated but do pass into milk in sufficient quantities to cause haemolytic anaemia in G6PD deficient babies (babies with a rare enzyme deficiency) or neonatal jaundice. Cautious use and careful observation is mandatory. Can also cause rashes.

Cotrimoxazole Not contra-indicated as amounts in breast milk are too small to have a significant action.

Tetracyclines Theoretically cause mottling of baby's developing teeth, though probably bound by calcium in breast milk, which retards absorption. Two authors recommend their avoidance by breast feeding mothers.

Penicillins Appear in trace amounts in breast milk and can cause allergic sensitization. Resulting levels in baby are not high enough to treat infections. An alternative antibiotic should ideally be used, though this may not always be possible.

Metronidazole According to manufacturer, the traces excreted in breast milk are harmless. Although carcinogenicity was reported in mice given this drug, this is not considered a contra-indication to its administration to the breast feeding mother now.

Nalidixic acid One case of haemolytic anaemia in baby whose mother was also taking amylobarbitone. Has also caused raised intracranial pressure. Use with caution if absolutely necessary and observe baby carefully.

Nitrofurantoin Level in breast milk not pharmacologically significant, but caution advised in G6PD deficient babies (babies with a rare enzyme deficiency).

Novobiocin Not recommended for breast feeding mothers because of possibility of neonatal jaundice.

Anticoagulants
Bleeding episodes have occurred after surgery or trauma in baby. Warfarin however is suitable for a breast feeding mother, as is heparin. Other drugs should be used with caution or substituted where possible with warfarin or heparin.

Cytotoxic drugs
Breast feeding is generally contra-indicated though one study concluded that methotrexate presented little hazard.

Antithyroid drugs
See also p. 165. One study concludes that they are not absolutely contra-indicated providing the dose is small and that the circulating thyroid hormones of the baby are closely monitored. The authors felt that propylthiouracil was the preferred drug for a breast feeding mother.

Central nervous system drugs

Alcohol See also p. 167. Can cause intoxication in the baby if large enough amounts are taken. Doses higher than 1g/kg of the mother's weight can inhibit the let down reflex, while doses higher than 2g/kg probably block it completely.

Amantadine Contra-indicated in the breast feeding mother, according to manufacturers, as it may cause vomiting, urinary retention and rashes in the baby.

Barbiturates Can cause drowsiness and may also stimulate the metabolism of other drugs taken by the mother. One case of cyanosis ('blue baby') due to methaemoglobinaemia occurred in a baby whose mother was also taking phenytoin.

Bromide Usually causes drowsiness and may cause a rash.

Carbamazepine Not advised by manufacturer if used in high doses or in combination with other antiepileptics, as there is a structural likeness to the tricyclics which are not metabolized in the young baby. However, no side-effects have actually been reported in the baby whose mother is taking the drug alone.

Chloral hydrate Can cause drowsiness in baby.

Chloroform Has been reported to cause deep sleep in baby.

Diazepam One report of lethargy and weight loss. Levels may build up in baby's body and cause neonatal jaundice. High doses are contra-indicated for the breast feeding mother.

Dichloralphenazone Causes slight drowsiness.

Heroin Can cause addiction in babies.

Lithium Baby should be carefully monitored for signs of lithium toxicity.

Morphine Significant amounts may be excreted in the milk of addicts.

Phenytoin One case of methaemoglobinaemia reported in baby whose mother was also taking phenobarbitone.

Tricyclic antidepressants According to one manufacturer, these are excreted in breast milk but are not metabolized in the young baby. This may theoretically result in accumulation. However, no side-effects in babies have been reported and it would seem safe for the breast feeding mother to take these provided the dose is not too high and the baby continues to thrive.

Sodium valproate The only report on this concludes that it is safe for the breast feeding mother to take.

Diuretics
Can decrease the milk supply.

Gastrointestinal drugs

Aloe Affected bowels of 12 out of 14 babies in one study.

Calomel Affected bowels of 7 out of 14 babies in one study.

Cascara Affected bowels of 10 out of 22 babies in one study.

Danthron Said by manufacturer to increase bowel activity in baby.

Phenolphthalein One study showed that the bowels of 16 out of 39 babies were affected, though two other studies showed no effect.

Senna Older senna preparations may affect baby's bowels but Senokot appears to have no effect in usual doses.

Hormones and synthetic substitutes

Corticosteroids (steroids) Studies in humans so far are inadequate but rat studies have produced death or growth retardation in sucklings after high daily doses. Most researchers advise against breast feeding.

Corticotrophin Said to increase the potassium and decrease the sodium in breast milk.

Sex hormones (including oral contraceptives) Oestrogen, oestrogen/progestogen and oestrogen/androgen combinations used in contraceptive doses can suppress lactation. Some studies have shown a decrease in protein, fat and minerals in breast milk. Isolated reports exist of breast enlargement in male babies, proliferation of the vaginal epithelium in female babies and changes in bones. One study, unconfirmed by others, showed a correlation between prior contraceptive use of these hormones and breast milk jaundice. Effects of progestogen-only pill on babies who are breast fed are not fully known as yet.

Miscellaneous drugs

Aspirin Large doses can cause rashes or gastrointestinal side-effects. Thought to be safe for mothers of breast-fed babies to take although it may be contra-indicated if the baby has a haematological or a clotting disorder.

Atropine Said to diminish milk flow and cause anticholinergic effects but no good documentation of this.

Bromocriptine Suppresses lactation. Prolactin levels fall within a few hours.

Digoxin Two recent reports conclude that even if the breast feeding mother is on a high dose of digoxin, the amounts secreted in breast milk are small and infant exposure is low.

Dihydrotachysterol Animal studies show decalcification of the bones. Some authors recommend that mothers taking this should not breast feed.

Ergometrine Lowers prolactin levels. It has been suggested that multiple doses might suppress lactation.

Ergot alkaloids 90 per cent of breast-fed babies had signs of ergotism (diarrhoea and vomiting; weak pulse; unstable blood pressure) in one study. Many derivatives can suppress lactation.

Gold Potential cause of rashes and other 'odd' reactions.

Hexachlorobenzene Many infant deaths in Turkey after mothers ate wheat treated with this insecticide.

Indomethacin Manufacturer recommends that this drug should not be given to a breast feeding mother. One case report of convulsions in a breast-fed baby whose mother took this drug.

Lead Lead toxicity (including encephalitis) has occurred after the use of lead acetate ointment on the nipples and after the use of lead breast shields.

Mercury Mothers exposed to high levels should not breast feed.

Nicotine May reduce milk supply. One case report of restlessness and circulatory disturbance. Smoking breast feeding mothers are more likely to give up breast feeding early than non-smokers.

Phenylbutazone Use with caution because of possible blood dyscrasias.

Pyridoxine One study showed a decrease in the milk supply.

Propanolol Only small amounts in milk of mothers taking this. However, because of the theoretical possibility of accumulation in the baby and because of the immaturity of enzyme systems responsible for metabolism, close observation for heart slowing or low blood sugar is necessary.

Reserpine One claim of significant nasal stuffiness and some increase in tracheobronchial secretions.

Radio-active drugs
Discard breast milk for a minimum of 24 hours, or until the milk is free of radio-activity, after a single dose. See also p. 165.

^{67}*Gallium citrate*[1] Significant amounts excreted in milk. Breast feeding contra-indicated.

^{125}*I labelled albumin*[2] Significant amounts excreted. Avoid the drug or stop breast feeding for at least 10 days.

^{131}*I*[2] Breast feeding contra-indicated after a large therapeutic dose. After smaller, diagnostic doses, discard milk for at least 24 hours (or for 72 hours, according to one author).

^{131}*I labelled macroaggregated albumin*[2] Discard breast milk for 10–12 days.

^{131}*I hippurate*[25] Discard breast milk for 24 hours.

^{99m}TCO_4[2] Discard breast milk for 32–72 hours.

^{99m}TCO_4 *labelled macroaggregated albumin*[1] Discard breast milk for 24 hours.

If you are going to have any radio-active isotope investigation or treatment don't forget to tell the doctor that you're breast feeding.

If your doctor would like to discuss any drug, the regional drug information centres, staffed by senior pharmacists, will be glad to help.

Questions and answers

Q Is it really necessary to eat more while breast feeding?
A Yes, it is. If you eat an extra 300–500 calories daily this still means that you're drawing on your own fat supplies to feed your baby, so if you didn't put on any extra fat during pregnancy and if you are fairly slim anyway, you will need to eat even more than this. In fact, the Department of Health in the UK currently recommends an extra 600 calories a day while breast feeding.

One survey found that stopping breast feeding because of 'not enough milk' was less likely in a group of mothers who had been actively encouraged to eat more, compared with a group who had had no such advice. Not all breast feeding mothers feel a need for extra food, though it's interesting that those who breast feed for longer tend to have larger appetites compared with their normal ones.

Q I am pregnant and breast feeding my first child, who is still taking quite a lot of milk from me. Will my next baby be deprived of the special benefits of colostrum when he is born because I am already producing mature milk?

A No one knows whether the large volumes of milk you are already making will be enriched by the extra antibodies, protein, zinc and other minerals, vitamins A, E, B_6 and B and live cells found in colostrum. However, this research is being started now. It seems highly unlikely that your baby would be at any disadvantage and certainly even mature breast milk would be better for him than cows' milk formula.

Q Could you say more about the feeding of a baby with a cleft lip and/or palate?

A (See also pp. 160–1.) Recommendations on breast feeding depend on the individual baby's condition and on the practice at the hospital. The Cleft Lip and Palate Association is undertaking an investigation into feeding techniques for these babies and may publish a leaflet giving general principles of feeding for parents. Their address is: The Hospital for Sick Children, Great Ormond Street, London, WC1N 3JH.

A dental plate sometimes called a 'pre-surgical appliance' or 'feeding plate' can be made for a baby with a cleft palate for use until the cleft is repaired. Each plastic plate is individually made from impressions taken of the baby's palate. It can be inserted as early as three days after birth and not only helps the baby to feed satisfactorily but also improves the alignment of the dental arches. Plates are made routinely at some hospitals and used only for severe clefts in others.

Different surgeons advise waiting for different lengths of time before the baby is allowed to suck after a cleft lip repair. Because of the danger of the scar splitting open, some suggest waiting for three to four weeks, while others allow sucking at ten days or even sooner. From both the baby's and the mother's points of view, the sooner sucking is started, the better, but obviously the healing of the scar takes first priority.

Q I had a Caesar and can't get comfortable feeding my baby lying down – is there a better way?
A If you have a horizontal scar, you can try sitting up, lying the baby on pillows on your lap and feeding in the usual way. With either a horizontal or a vertical scar, try sitting up and lying the baby on a pillow with his head facing the breast and his legs tucked under your arm on that side. Alternatively, with you sitting up, lie him on a pillow at your side with his legs across your thighs and support his head either with another pillow at the correct length or with your arm, in turn supported by a pillow. The point of all these positions is to take the weight of the baby off your abdomen and to avoid the strain on your abdominal muscles of holding the baby to your breast. Sit straight to avoid straining your abdomen.

Q My baby spends a large amount of time during a feed just holding the nipple in his mouth without sucking. Is this normal?
A Yes. It's partly caused by your let-down pattern (see pp. 24–5) but one researcher has also noted that 'newborn infants write their signature with their sucking rhythm, showing a constant, individual pattern in the number of sucks and intervals between sucks per minute'. This also helps explain why some babies take longer over a feed than others.

Q I've tried everything but my baby still cries in the early evening and isn't satisfied at the breast. Is there anything else I can do?
A It's been suggested by some experts that the milk supply may fall in the late afternoon and early evening if you don't have anything to eat between lunch time and supper time. Many women give their babies several feeds without thinking of feeding

themselves to 'make the milk'. Try making it a habit to have something to eat between each of your baby's feeds.

Q My friend says my milk doesn't look rich enough for my baby because it's bluish-white. What do you think?
A This is the normal colour of breast milk in many women, though you'll probably notice that the colour of your milk is different at the beginning and end of a feed and this colour difference depends on its fat content. We're more used to the colour of cows' milk, but that doesn't make it a 'better' colour than breast milk and certainly doesn't mean that it is in any way more suitable for babies.

Q Is there any evidence that babies can recognize their mother's milk?
A The answer to this is complicated. Studies in France and England have found that a baby turns to a pad that has been placed next to his mother's breast in preference to a clean one which has neither breast milk on it nor has been in contact with the breast. Further experiments have shown that it is the breast contact that is most important because babies don't turn to pads soaked in their mother's expressed breast milk.

Just what it is on the mother's breast that produces this unique recognition is not known but it could be a smell, caused, for example, by natural chemicals called pheromones which are hormone-like substances known to be vital in animal recognition systems. Many mothers say they can recognize their babies by smell alone but there is as yet no hard evidence on this.

Q Considering that diabetes is such a common problem, I wonder if you could give more information about diabetic mothers and breast feeding?
A Diabetes certainly is a common condition, affecting as it does about 2 per cent of the population, but because so few women choose to breast feed, research into the effects on a diabetic mother and her baby is scanty. In one American study, 17 breast-feeding, insulin-dependent diabetic mothers were followed, 14 of whom fed their babies for more than nine

months. Several useful tips came out of their experiences. High motivation and unusual support from family, friends and health professionals meant that all these women were able to breast feed successfully. Care is especially necessary if baby and mother are separated after delivery. Frequent expression of milk, or, preferably, visits to the baby for him to be cuddled and put to the breast are essential to work up the milk supply.

About 5–7 hours after delivery there is an increased risk of the mother's blood sugar becoming too low (hypoglycaemia) since the loss of the hormone placental lactogen is accompanied by an increased sensitivity to insulin. This happens whether or not a mother is breast feeding, and as soon as diet-insulin-exercise adjustments are made, the blood sugar stabilizes. Most mothers find that during the first 4–6 weeks, their insulin requirement is less than before they became pregnant. Breast feeding itself may reduce the insulin requirement for longer than this period. Four women in the survey, however, needed more insulin during the first three months after delivery than before they became pregnant, probably because they were eating more and exercising less.

Hypoglycaemic (insulin) reactions cause the release of adrenalin which decreases the blood flow through the arteries in the breasts and can also inhibit the let-down reflex. Traces of insulin and adrenalin pass into the milk but are inactivated by the baby's digestive enzymes.

Infections should always be treated quickly in diabetics and the antibiotic chosen must be safe for the breast-fed baby. Diabetic women are more prone to monilial ('thrush') infection of the vagina which can spread to affect the nipples. The nipples should be kept dry to help prevent this happening.

Breast-fed babies may suddenly want either more or less frequent feeds, perhaps because of illness or a growth spurt. This can cause unexpectedly low or high blood sugar levels in diabetic mothers, levels which can be compensated for by adjusting the diet, exercise and insulin dose.

Q I have hyperprolactinaemia. Should I breast feed?

A Infertility caused by hyperprolactinaemia can often be

successfully treated with a drug called bromocriptine. This lowers the blood prolactin level and enables conception to occur. Once you've got your baby though, the drug can't be used to keep the prolactin low if you want to breast feed, because it dries the milk up!

Because breast feeding raises the blood prolactin level further, women are discouraged from doing it for two reasons. First there seems to be five times the risk of getting a breast abscess and, second, a sizeable proportion of women with this condition have a tumour of the pituitary gland. Raising the prolactin level by breast feeding could lead to an increase in the size of such a tumour. Because of the position of the tumour, enlargement can lead to visual disturbances, including blindness.

If the raised prolactin levels of pregnancy have not already led to an increase in size of a woman's tumour (as gauged by visual field measurements and special x-rays), and if she is particularly keen to breast feed, a woman could have regular checks of her visual fields and regular x-rays so that she could stop breast feeding at the first suspicion of any increase in tumour size. These tests are, however, time-consuming for the woman and expensive for the health service.

Q Is it true that vegans and vegetarians cannot produce good quality milk and so should not breast feed their babies?

A We really need to consider these two groups of people separately because their diets are very different from a breast-feeding point of view. Vegetarians usually eat some eggs, cheese, fish and foods other than vegetables, contrary to popular belief. Because of this their intake of vitamin B_{12} is usually adequate and does not need supplementing during everyday life, pregnancy or while breast feeding. As far as we know, the breast milk of vegetarians is also perfectly healthy in other respects and interestingly contains high levels of polyunsaturated fatty acids. The implications of this are not clear.

Vegans eat no animal foods at all and are therefore at risk of being short of vitamin B_{12}, essential for the normal formation of red blood cells and the normal functioning of nervous tissue. Vegans must take vitamin B_{12} both during pregnancy and when breast feeding and some experts think they should take it all the time anyway. Studies have shown that when a vegan mother's diet is supplemented with this vitamin, her milk contains normal amounts of vitamin B_{12} and her baby is perfectly safe.

Q Must I have a nursing bra? Couldn't I make do with a good ordinary one?

A (See also pp. 72–3.) Very many women manage perfectly well without nursing bras and find that it is far easier simply to pull the cup of an ordinary bra down, rather than fiddling with the hooks of nursing bras. It'll obviously be easier to do this if your bra is soft, elastic and not too built-up.

Q From the way you describe the expression of breast milk it seems that you have to keep your hand in the same position throughout. Is this so?

A No. When expressing your milk (see p. 96), it's important to express it from all parts of the breast. You will need to move your thumb and finger to several different positions to do this, and to use your other hand if necessary.

If you are expressing milk after you've fed your baby, perhaps because you want to leave breast milk in the fridge for a baby sitter to give your baby, don't be put off by the small amounts of milk which appear. The fractions of an ounce soon mount up if you collect after each feed for a couple of days in advance of needing it.

Q Do I need to take extra vitamin D if I'm breast feeding?

A We now know that sunshine is a far better source of vitamin D than any food. Vitamin D produced in the skin after exposure to sunlight can be stored and used during the winter months. It makes sense for the woman who is pregnant or breast feeding to get as much sun as she can and for babies to be allowed to sunbathe when possible, taking care to avoid overexposure. (See also pp. 38 and 192.)

Although sunshine is the most important source of vitamin D. it's sensible to ensure that your diet during pregnancy and breast feeding includes plenty of vitamin D-containing foods (margarine, fatty fish, eggs and butter). For mothers who have little exposure to sunlight or whose diets are deficient in this vitamin, vitamin D supplements are available.

Q Can my baby's colic really be caused by cows' milk in my breast milk?

A A recent study from Sweden suggests that this is likely. Twelve out of nineteen colicky breast-fed babies lost their colic when their mothers were put on a diet free from cows' milk protein. The colic reappeared on at least two further 'challenges' (in the form of a diet containing cows' milk for the mother). At four months, only four of the babies reacted with colic when their mothers had cows' milk in their diets, which fits in well with the observation that most babies tend to lose their colic after three or four months anyway. We know that whole molecules of cows' milk protein (and other dietary proteins) can be present in breast milk, and we know that colic is a well recognized symptom of cows' milk protein intolerance, so the theory could well be right.

There is a suggestion that breast-fed babies might benefit from exposure to 'foreign' proteins and other dietary substances in breast milk, because it helps prepare their immunity system gradually for the switch to a mixed diet. However, certain babies – the colicky ones included – may be unable to cope with these food traces in breast milk and this inability to cope may be more likely if there is an allergic family history.

Some allergy experts suggest that the breast feeding mother of a child with an allergic family history, or just with colic, should vary her diet so as to avoid a large intake of any one specific food, particularly cows' milk. Eggs, bananas, apples, oranges, strawberries, tomatoes, coffee and chocolate have also been associated with colic in the breast-fed baby if the mother has too much of them.

Q Is it all right for me to breast feed my friend's baby if he cries while he has been left with me?

A There's no reason why you shouldn't, and it'll save her having to express milk to leave in a bottle for you to give him.

Make sure your own baby gets enough, though! Wet nursing each other's babies is on the increase. One day we may even see a return to the old fashioned and formerly widely accepted practice of wet nursing, with baby minders offering such a service.

Q My newborn baby doesn't ask for many feeds and isn't putting on enough weight. What should I do?
A Your baby needs to be fed more often, so put him to the breast at least twice as frequently. The stimulus to your breasts from more frequent feeds will increase your milk supply over a few days. Don't cut short the length of the feeds but let him suck for as long as he wants to. Some babies like to suck on and off for long periods, perhaps falling asleep every few minutes, and only start taking more 'formal' feeds when they are older and stronger.

Some babies need to be reminded that the breast is there before they ask for feeds and the smell of your skin and milk can help to do this. Other feeding stimuli are the sounds your body makes – your voice, heartbeats and tummy rumbles, the sight of you and the feel of you. A baby left lying alone in his cot only has the stimulus of his empty tummy to remind him of you and your breasts, and this isn't always enough, especially if he is of low birth weight, jaundiced, ill, or apathetic following the use of pethidine during your labour. Keep your disinterested baby with you as much as possible, either lying in your arms as you sit up, lying beside you as you sit or lie in bed, or in your arms or a sling as you do things. All the stimuli he'll receive from you will encourage him to ask for and to be alert enough to take the breast more often.

Q You give the impression that breast feeding involves feeding the baby very frequently for months on end. Is this right?
A Babies are all different and some want more frequent feeding than others. During the early days, most mothers find that their babies settle better on frequent feeds. If your baby wants frequent feeds, you soon get used to it. Feeds become second nature and not big occasions to plan for. As they grow older,

many babies ask for fewer feeds and some settle into their own individual 'routines' which may happen by chance to be roughly 2, 3 or 4 hourly feeds.

Sometimes you may find that your baby will want feeding much more often than usual. He may be extra hungry because he's growing fast; because he's ill, teething, or just upset. If he needs more milk, your milk supply will catch up in two or three days if you let him feed as much as he wants. If not, just letting him have unrestricted access to your breast will soothe him. Mothers who put their babies to the breast as often as the babies want to usually feed much more often than schedule feeders. Their feeds also seem more effortless because they are taken so much in their stride.

Q Are breast-fed babies less likely to get nappy rash?
A Yes. The stools of a breast-fed baby are more acid than those of a bottle-fed one because of the presence in the bowels of bacteria (see p. 39) which produce acetic and lactic acids. The commonest type of nappy rash, ammonia dermatitis, is caused by the release of ammonia from urea in urine by certain bacteria in the stools. This is much more likely to happen if the stools are alkaline, as in bottle-fed babies.

Q My baby has suddenly started fighting at the breast at three months. Can you help?
A It sounds as though your baby may be frustrated because you don't have enough milk. Three months is a common time for the supply to dwindle, usually because of insufficient stimulation of the breasts by too few feeds. Try increasing your milk supply by feeding him much more often and for as long as he wants to suck. He should be happier within two or three days. (See also pp. 154–5.)

If your baby sleeps through the night, this may be jeopardizing your supply as your breasts are unemptied for too long. Wake your baby to feed him or express some milk when you go to bed and if you wake up during the night with tense breasts. Waking the baby is more efficient and quicker than expressing.

Q I'm taking breast milk to the hospital each day for my baby who's in the special care baby unit, but I haven't a fridge. How should I store the milk?

A Buy two ice packs (from a camping shop) and leave one at the hospital each day to be refrozen. At home, keep the bottle of milk with a frozen ice pack on top in a closed, insulated container such as a freezer bag or a polystyrene picnic box, or even simply a cardboard box lined thickly with newspaper. Keep the container in the coldest place you can find; and use it for carrying the milk to the hospital too.

Q Why are there no references in your book to the scientific literature that you so widely quote from?

A We did consider having a bibliography but an exhaustive list of all the research and review papers, books and other sources we used would fill almost half of the book! A selected reference list would have left out too many small but interesting sources of information to be acceptable.

Index